On Diagnosis:

A Systemic Approach

On Diagnosis

A Systemic Approach

By

Michael L. Glenn, M.D.

BRUNNER/MAZEL, *Publishers* • New York

Library of Congress Cataloging in Publication Data

Glenn, Michael L. (Michael Lyon), 1938-
   On diagnosis.

   Bibliography: p.
   Includes index.
   1. Medicine, Psychosomatic. 2. Diagnosis—Social
aspects. I. Title. [DNLM: 1. Diagnosis. 2. Family
practice. 3. Physician—Patient relations.
4. Psychosomatic medicine. WB 141 G55080]
RC49.G566   1984   616.07'5'01   84-7095
ISBN 0-87630-361-0

Copyright © 1984 by Michael L. Glenn

Published by
Brunner/Mazel, Inc.
19 Union Square West
New York, New York 10003

MANUFACTURED IN THE UNITED STATES OF AMERICA

To my family.

Contents

III. NOSOLOGICAL AND OTHER QUESTIONS

Preface

This book emerged out of a clinical dilemma I often face as a family practitioner, the dilemma of figuring out what is "really" wrong with the person who has come to me for care, and what to do about it. Reflecting on my daily activity, I realized that some of my work is ridiculously easy, but most of it is very hard. It is easy when people come in for a shot, or with a sore throat, a cough, or a sprained foot. It is hard most of the rest of the time.

Here are the kind of things that make me scratch my head with frustration:

1) People come in with persistent physical complaints which I cannot explain.
2) People come in for a general physical exam, and seem healthy; yet they are obviously laboring under a lot of stress and worry.
3) People come in because of some physical complaint which appears almost certainly related to anxiety or depression, but they refuse to admit being either anxious or depressed.
4) People come in with several different medical problems, but also appear worried, preoccupied, and upset with events happening in their lives; further, the interplay of these two, though apparently of great significance, is difficult to grasp.
5) People come in with distressing symptoms of significant diseases,

but I am struck by how fanatically obsessed they are with these diseases and their symptoms.

6) People come in, apparently wanting to be pronounced healthy; but when this is done they become upset and appear to want some clear-cut physical illness instead, which could "explain" their distress to them and to their families.

7) People come in repeatedly for medical appointments, but it is not clear to me why they come, why they keep coming back, and what they want from me: It is as if I am supposed to discover why they continue seeking my attention.

And this is just the beginning of the "hard" part.

I am not sure how to express this dilemma. It is as if the medical encounter, a particular permissible form of human encounter, is being used as a context for different scripts and agendas. Ostensibly, the encounter has a "medical" basis. Two people do not simply come together and chat—their interaction is supposed to focus on a problem which one of them (the patient) brings to the other (the physician). And yet, I keep feeling that this is only a fraction of the story.

In this basic encounter between people, I find myself again and again wanting to ask: "So tell me, how is it with you in your life now?" Some of the time this question seems wholly inappropriate; other times it seems exactly what the patient has wanted me to say.

My problem got harder, because I realized I didn't always have the time to ask such a question, to respond to an answer, or to explain why I might want to ask it when the patient came to the office with some other agenda.

Also, I realized that in the medical relationship, as in many other relationships, one cannot wholly satisfy one's own agenda: Questions remain unasked, hunches remain unspoken, curiosity remains unsatisfied. I simply cannot know everything I might want to know about my patients. After all, I don't let them in on everything I myself am coping with, thinking, and feeling about my own state of "being in the world."

So what, I wondered, is happening? How was I to answer the simplest of questions, like, "What's wrong with this patient?" or "Why is this patient coming in month after month, and what can I do about it?"

Reflecting on this problem, I began realizing that it emerged out of the nature of medical (primary care) practice. Like other physicians, I was trained to look for pathology, to group a patient's symptoms into some recognizable disease pattern or else to proclaim them a "non-disease" and the patient "healthy." I also had the added benefit of psychiatric training, which had taught me to understand people's different styles of being in the world, different ways of experiencing it, and different ways of presenting themselves to others. This took the form of character typology (MacKinnon and Michels, 1971) more than any ubiquitous organized psychopathology; but I had been trained in the latter, too.

Yet such training did not prepare me for understanding what was "wrong" with the people who came to me for treatment. It helped me grasp a slice of "what was wrong," but it didn't help me get my hands around the whole thing.

Let me give you a picture of two or three patients that create such problems. First, a lengthy example:

Annie Y, a 61-year-old woman, initially came to me requesting weekly vitamin B-12 shots. A previous physician had given this to her, and she now felt she "needed" it. She also complained of being "nervous." Physical exam showed that she had a blood pressure of 160/106; her cardiogram showed evidence of an old heart attack, and some signs that she was not getting enough blood to the vessels serving her heart muscle. Otherwise her physical exam was normal.

She was divorced. She had no children. She lived close to her mother, who had been depressed for years and who weighed close to 300 pounds, and a sister who had suffered several psychotic episodes of depression. She constantly worried about her health. "Is my heart bad? Oh God, is it *serious*? Why do I feel so tired? What makes my arms ache? Are you sure I don't have arthritis?" She denied having any past heart attack.

I obtained a stress test, which was normal. I prescribed nitrates for her heart, but she refused to take them. I prescribed a medley of antihypertensive medications, but all of them "made her sick," and she refused to take them. She did take a sedative, but her blood pressure did not really come down, and we embarked on a course of trying to find an acceptable antihypertensive program.

She came weekly, insisting on B-12 shots. She talked to a therapist once, and pronounced it a waste of time. My view of her was 1) a hypochondriacally obsessed woman, 2) chronically depressed, 3) who had suffered a silent heart attack some time in the past and who was therefore "at risk," and 4) who still suffered from hypertension.

But this description does not do justice to the interaction. This woman and I were in different worlds, on totally different wavelengths. She would ask a question, I would answer it, and it was as if my answer had never been said. Her obsessive worrying knew no bounds. It could not be answered directly. And any attempt to deal with it on a meta-level was stymied by her refusal to deal with the emotional aspects of her life, and instead to ask repeatedly about her physical health.

Next, a smaller example:

Sammy P, an eight-year-old boy, kept being dragged in by his mother with somatic complaints. When he came in, she would say he was having trouble. He would deny it. The two of them would fight. He would grudgingly admit his symptoms. Examination would be negative. I would give him a minor placebo. The mother would deny any other problems in the house, other than a little "stress" which she preferred not to discuss further. Following two or three weeks, the boy would improve; but I would see him again six months later for something else.

A final example should make this even clearer:

Helen B is an elderly woman with bowel dysfunction. She comes and talks to me about her constipation and diarrhea, every two weeks. She also gets placebo B-12 shots. If I ask her to come in at lengthier intervals, she does not argue. She simply gets "sick" before her appointment comes, and winds up coming in every two weeks anyway. If I do not take blood tests when she feels she wants them, or a yearly EKG which I have told her is unnecessary, she develops severe chest pain or some other symptom which categorically demands that I do those tests. She will not talk to me about other events in her life. There's "nothing to talk about." She denies depression. She denies wanting to see me every two weeks. Yet my perception is that she is somatically fixated on her bowels and that she parlays this into regular sessions with me, which are somehow helpful to her, and which she tenaciously will not give up.

As I took on my patients' day-to-day complaints, I found myself more and more perplexed, stymied trying to figure out just what was going on. What was the "real problem" people were trying to present?

I turned to the writings of medical sociologists whose perspective on the doctor-patient relationship closely resembled my own. These authors discussed the diverse social and cultural, as well as personal, influences on the medical encounter. They clarified such common factors as the patient's intent and concerns, the physician's training and bias, the social roles the encounter serves to further, and its economic basis. I tried to understand my dilemma in a more organized way.

The problem crystalized for me around the question of diagnosis. Diagnosis describes "what's going on." Yet traditional texts on diagnosis keep the medical encounter confined to the search for a physical or mental "disease." They narrow the focus and deprive it of richer meanings and context.

Then I reread Michael Balint's work on *The Doctor, His Patient, and the Illness* (1957). I realized that Balint was taking physical illness and putting it into an interpersonal, psychological context, much as sociologists like Freidson had put it into its social and cultural context. Balint was looking much more deeply into the medical encounter, trying to get at its reason for existence, at the motives behind both patient's and physician's being there. His discussion of the different "levels" of diagnosis illuminated my own dilemma. Here I was, trying to get a handle on the emotional context in which a patient's symptoms were presented, wanting to deal with the whole patient. My problem had often become painfully clear when, trying to pursue a "deeper" level, I encountered sharp resistance from the patient, who insisted instead on pursuing the physical dimensions only.

Let me put it this way. Suppose that people are basically physically ill (with some problem or another, or several) or physically healthy. Suppose that they are neurotic in their concerns (as evaluated by someone observing them) or appropriately concerned. Suppose that bodily symptoms are brought about both by physical abnormalities and by emotional tension (or other causes). Now consider the confusion and uncertainty this set of givens has created.

Here we have a person who appears to be neurotic and worried, complaining endlessly about somatic problems, but "physically well." There we have the exact same person, with the exact same personality pattern and complaints, but with a severe, life-threatening disease. And over there is a person with the exact same complaints and life-threatening disease, but with no apparent "neurotic" underpinnings at all, and who on the contrary appears quite appropriate in her interaction with the medical system.

Furthermore, physicians differ from one another; and one physician and a patient can differ so strongly that they seem to be talking "two different languages" when they meet.

What then?

The more I thought about it, the more I felt that the physician's initial and fundamental task was to describe "what's going on"—in all its complexity. This is diagnosis. It may be simple or it may be complex. It may be a strep throat in a 24-year-old man (simple) or repetitive belly pains in a tense 11-year-old girl (complex); its treatment may be simple or complex, too, perhaps more than a matter of simply prescribing a bottle of green medicine to be taken *ad lib.*

One of the earliest and one of the most serious influences on my thinking was the maverick psychiatrist Thomas Szasz. His critique of "mental illness" brought an appreciation of the social role of psychiatry and psychiatrists into that field, and forced an entire generation of psychiatrists (myself included at that time) to consider the social context of what they did. Michael Balint's accomplishment, though not at all similar on the surface of things, was in some way a parallel act. Balint was attempting to demolish the easy myth of "physical illness," much as Szasz devastated the easy notion of "mental illness."

Szasz had claimed that psychiatrists were inappropriately labeling deviant or unusual behavior as a "mental illness"—to which his conclusion was: This is nonsense. Perhaps this is ethics or politics or religion, but it is not medicine. Medicine is concerned with real physical illnesses, and bizarre behavior is no proof of anything like that.

Szasz claimed there was only one kind of illness: physical illness, pure and simple. But this was just what I was finding so difficult to deal with in actual practice. Balint provided an answer, for he pointed out how physicians (and others) were always trying to find "physical illnesses" in everything, often to the detriment of the patient's own experience. Balint implies that coming to a physician's office is no proof that one is sick, even though the physician may proceed as if it were. Here is the comparison. Neither conventional psychiatry nor conventional medicine is prepared to probe beneath the surface of their patients' problems, to seek meaning in the pattern, to situate the part in the context of the whole. Whereas Szasz would claim that this is "beyond" the realm of medicine, Balint argues that these other realms are absolutely germane, and that they constitute a challenge to the thinking physician.

I then understood what I had liked and had not liked in Szasz, and sensed that, although physical illness might indeed "exist," defining it was often not the main problem with which the practitioner had to cope. I was beginning to get my hands around the problem.

These thoughts are the basic goad towards my writing the book you're now holding in your hands. None of the texts I looked at came close to providing an adequate, satisfactory explanation of the process and import of diagnosis. Bits of understanding appeared scattered over the intellectual universe: Balint, Szasz, the medical sociologists, the family systems thinkers, the old-time GP's, the new family practitioners. I felt it was important to bring these different threads together and try to weave them into a single fabric.

One further ingredient shaped my thinking in this matter. This was the increasing role of what has come to be called a systems way of looking at the world. Systems theory provides a theoretical framework capable of handling the different pieces involved in a phenomenon like the medical encounter. It can deal with elements from different "systems" and with their interaction. It can deal with differences at the individual level, at the family level, and at the level of peer group, cultural or ethnic group, community, and so on. In other words, the breadth of systems theory provides a time/space grid with collapsible eye-pieces, which can describe the different factors involved in an event like diagnosis better than any other available framework.

Systems theory arose initially in the physical sciences, and then moved into the social sciences. Gradually, cautiously, it has crept into medicine. Perhaps the most influential writer in this regard has been George Engel. Engel has been writing about the need for a new medical model for the past 20 years. He has popularized diagrams which show the hierarchy and continuum of systems, for example, and he has over and over tried to show how such a theory can help physicians look at the patient's body at the organ-system level, at the organ level, and even at cellular, humoral, biochemical, and immunological levels.

I had tended to view behavior from the standpoint of individual (or marital/family) psychodynamics. Now I was beginning to appreciate the broader determinants of how people felt and of what they said and did. I felt it was time to put down what I had understood so others could use it.

I have written this book at a level which should be able to explain its basic concepts to the medical student, the student of medical sociology, or the practicing family physician. I hope one of the book's main uses will be in medical schools, to help future doctors appreciate how complicated the diagnostic process is. Certainly, I am not proposing new answers for the problem of medical diagnosis. But I am trying to keep practitioners from prematurely closing off vast areas which affect the meaning of symptoms, the purpose of the medical encounter, and the "illness" as it operates in context.

My plan for the book is very simple. I begin with an examination of how the problem presents itself to the practitioner, and give a compact account of how this came to be so (Introduction). Then, after a clinical example which portrays the dilemma I have alluded to already (Chapter 1), I begin an analysis of the diagnostic process. This begins with a discussion of the traditional view of diagnosis and some critiques of it (Chapters 2 and 3).

The next several chapters go more in depth into some of the basic aspects of the diagnostic process. Chapter 4 looks at the context in which diagnosis occurs, the intersection of the medical system and the family system. Chapter 5 examines how the diagnosis actually takes place, interactionally. Chapter 6 considers the question, What disease is being diagnosed? Chapter 7 looks further at diagnosis as knowledge or hypothesis.

The second section of the book looks at the many different kinds of diagnostic contracts which occur in medical practice. I hope their clarity and diversity give the reader a graphic understanding of the dilemma I'm discussing.

Finally, a brief third section addresses the problem of nosology and classification today.

If I succeed in making the reader a bit more hesitant and uncertain about traditional notions of diagnosis, I will be pleased.

Many people have helped me develop the ideas in this book. I should like to thank some of them by name: Lucy Candib and Ron Ransom, kindred spirits whose stimulating talk and warm personal support have been important to me; Don Bloch and Barry Dym, whose unvarying systems perspective has often served to correct my medical excesses; Janet Christie-Seely, Mac Baird, Roger Bibace, and Don Cassata, whose dedication towards a systems perspective in family medicine has been undaunted. I am also indebted to people who live for me through their books; the network of ideas has made me their unknown friend and admirer: George Engel, Eliot Freidson, John Stoeckle, Eliot Mishler and the late Michael Balint. Finally, I owe much to my colleagues in the Everett Family Practice, Linda Atkins and Robert Singer (without whose being on call half the time, this book would never have been written): Our weekly conversations have helped sharpen my own ideas, and I'm sure have given me some of theirs.

M.L.G.

Introduction

Establishing a diagnosis is one of the physician's most basic tasks. Without diagnosis, treatment is haphazard, lacking in scientific basis, and impossible to evaluate. Diagnosis brings pattern to the patient's random complaints and organizes symptoms into a meaningful gestalt. It creates illness as a recognizable thing, an entity which goes beyond the patient's subjective sensation of being sick; thus, it paves the way to rational treatment. Without diagnosis, the practitioner is left to struggle with individual symptoms one by one, without an overarching plan; and the patient is left with a raggle-taggle assortment of worrisome symptoms which do not appear to make sense.

Diagnosis has further implications. It is not just an *idea*, a *concept*. It is a vital criterion which affects the organization and functioning of the entire health care system. In this age of third-party payment, diagnosis determines which services will be reimbursed and which will not; which health care providers will be paid, and which will not; which patients will receive disability compensation, and which will not. In the "old days," a physician may have kept his records in his head, but now that will not suffice. Records must be available for review. Data must be tabulated. Charts must be up-to-date. The diagnosis must be on the "encounter form" which describes the patient's visit, and that diagnosis will determine if money flows into a major hospital, a physician's office, a teaching center, or a local clinic; and, if so, how much.

The currently used notions of diagnosis, however, are grounded in 19th-century perspectives. They rely on morbid anatomy, which explains illness on the basis of diseased body parts, or on morbid physiology, which explains illness on the basis of malfunctioning body systems. Such notions distort the breadth of what we have learned about sickness today. They force us to cram our understanding into much narrower channels than they belong, and often make the diagnostic process arbitrary and incomplete. Each time we use the principles of diagnosis this way, we do a disservice to the patient being considered, to the process we are trying to describe, to the principles of science itself, and to ourselves as thinking beings.

The notion of one illness, one cause, one process, one treatment no longer corresponds to the reality of most "illnesses" today. Yet this is how they are usually discussed. This is how they must be named, because this is how they appear in the Nomenclature of Disease and in the insurance diagnostic codebooks. This is how they have been considered for most research work, as well as for most medical care. In spite of much contemporary rhetoric about treating the whole person and viewing illnesses in context, most actual medical practice is too rigidly bound to incorporate such a perspective. Even if physicians wanted to expand their scope, few third parties would pay them for their time or effort. Traditional notions of diagnosis, bolstered by the medical system they have helped shape, perpetuate a fragmented understanding of health care and lead to its natural consequence—the fragmented, specialist-based organization of services.

Twentieth-century notions of diagnosis were based upon the medical model of disease dating from the latter part of the 19th century. This positivistic model was built upon the doctrine of the specific etiology of disease, which sought to explain each illness by a specific causative agent. Once the offending agent was identified, rational treatment could begin. In this model illness was *real*: It existed "out there" and could be apprehended by objective, scientific tests. It was also *universal*: Tuberculosis, for example, could be treated the same way, no matter who happened to contract the disease, where they lived, how old they were, and so on. The main problem was simply diagnosing the illness: All else followed from this first step.

Diagnosis was the consummate task of the skilled physician—an astute act of inductive reasoning, which embraced clinical acumen, scholarly prowess, judgment, and intuition. It was like the entomologist's identifying a new and complicated insect: First, he carefully studies its diverse attributes; then he refers his findings to some "fixed" classification schema; finally he pins the correct label on his object of study. Diagnosis was a similarly scientific and intellectual feat.

This notion worked well for decades, especially in regard to the infectious diseases. It offered great promise in approaching diseases caused by genetic abnormalities, too; and, for a time, seemed capable of describing even the large number of complicated illnesses involving many systems, by pointing out the one "basic" biochemical or genetic flaw.

But this "biomedical" model began to break down when it came to explaining the diseases which affect millions of people today—those whose etiology seems unclear, multifactored, and stress-related. Coronary artery disease, asthma, diabetes, the collagen diseases, and cancers—most of the commonly occurring diseases—are not well understood today. They overwhelm the biomedical model whenever it attempts to explain them. For example, millions of people suffer from hypertension, but physicians cannot agree what level of blood pressure reading defines the disease. (Is it a diastolic of more than 90mm or 95mm?) Furthermore, physicians disagree on whether treatment of low grade hypertension affects the course of the disease. And if treatment does affect the disease, physicians disagree about which forms of treatment are best. Finally, physicians are not sure what the main cause of "idiopathic" hypertension is, how it develops, and so on. Especially unclear is the role of "stress" in causing the disease—compared, say, to the role of salt metabolism—and what to do about it.

Peptic ulcer disease would be another common example. This very common illness is poorly understood. "Stress" is felt to be important in its development, yet psychological factors are not dealt with in the usual diagnostic categories of the disease, which only deal with the type of ulcer, its location, whether it is recurrent, and so on.

Because of advances in today's depth of understanding about the divers factors which can affect a given disease like hypertension or peptic ulcer, the linear cause-and-effect model of 19th-century diagnostics feels grossly inadequate. Yet this is all that is currently available.

The medical model has been amended as if it were the U.S. Constitution. It is now capable of handling not just one but a multitude of simultaneous, causative factors, consistent with the progress in medical knowledge. This reflects our understanding that many coexisting factors may affect a disease process. *Genetic* factors predispose to many illnesses, as well as constituting the main cause of certain syndromes. *Host* factors are far more complex than was earlier thought: Exposure to the same offending agent may produce an illness in some people but not in others, depending on host resistance; and host resistance itself, bound up in the integrity of the immune system, may vary day by day, depending on a diversity of factors. Furthermore, the offending *agent* may vary, too; and *environmental factors*, such as air pollution, noise level, exposure to toxins at work, etc., may play a critical role in the development of disease. Finally, *social and emotional factors* have now been shown to be crucial co-determinants of the disease process, and they must be considered, too.

As if this were not enough, the interplay between these different forces is itself a variable factor in the appearance of disease. Sophisticated research has yielded new information about interconnections between psychosocial and physical factors in health and disease, and it is clear that host resistance and susceptibility to disease are extremely complex. Interaction between stressors and host responses influences the outbreak, the severity, and the course of disease. An individual capable of warding off an illness at one time may not be able to cope with it as effectively a few weeks later. People change; and as they change, their resistance to disease changes, too. Diseases change, too. Beyond this, there appear to be some random factors which defy the positivist outlook, and which can only be handled by reference to a stochastic model of disease, and by an epidemiological, not a personal, approach.

Perceiving this, the biomedical model initially struggled to adapt. Theories of disease were amended to include a complexity of involved factors. Simple notions of mechanical causality gave way to views of stages, "necessary causes" and "precipitating causes," and so on. But this was not enough. The model was already beginning to crumble. A new model was sought (Engel, 1977), which could explore illness in the broader context more consistent with the scope of our understanding.

Earlier tradition had, of course, appreciated illness in a much broader context. Socrates had commented that "there is no disease of the body apart from the soul." Hippocrates is famous for his counsel that the physician should be familiar with the physical and social environment of his patient:

> A physician must know . . . what man is in relation to foods and drinks, and to habits generally, and [to] what will be the effects of each on each individual. . . . (pp. 53, 55)
> Whoever wishes to pursue properly the science of medicine must . . . consider what effects each season of the year can produce . . . the hot winds and the cold . . . the properties of the

waters . . . the soil, too . . . the mode of life of the inhabitants. . . .
(p. 71)

In fact, until well into the 19th century, the prevailing model of medical thought was much closer to what we today would call "holistic" than it was to the germ theory of disease.

In contemporary thought, Auerswald (1968, 1983) has described the "ecology" of illness, and a growing trend has preoccupied itself with investigating the broader context in which illness occurs. Many general practitioners have made observations along this line in the past four decades (cf. Huygen, 1982; Kellner, 1963; Richardson, 1948); and other insights have come from social scientists investigating "deviant" behavior (Antonovsky, 1979; Segall, 1976; Twaddle, 1972) and from the various therapy fields.

The question of illness itself was opened up to examination when Szasz (1974) challenged the application of the biomedical model to psychiatry and denounced the "myth of mental illness." Others doubted that "illnesses" like alcoholism, depression, or hyperactivity actually existed. Illich (1976) decried the medicalization of American society, through which medical labels were applied to a number of normative processes, moral or legal issues, and political conflicts; he pointed out how this process stripped many human activities of their deeper significance and turned them into medical events, thus elevating the physician into the position of authority in many areas of living that physicians knew very little about.

But while ferment in some circles over these issues was becoming intense, medicine as a whole seemed only to be deepening its commitment to the biomedical model, both as a didactic tool and as a way of organizing clinical practice. Medical students were strongly encouraged to become specialists. Technology mushroomed, bringing even greater specialization in its wake. Status and respect were accorded to the physicians who had mastered the most recent tests and techniques. Research became more and more fragmented. The generalists were viewed as a vanishing breed. Whereas 84% of physicians in the 1930s had been GP's, by 1966, 84% had become specialists.

An alternative paradigm arose when George Engel put forth his "biopsychosocial" model of illness (1977). This model introduced a systemic approach into general medicine, and it currently serves as a rallying point for a growing number of physicians and other health practitioners interested in moving beyond the biomedical model of disease. In recent years the professional base for the advocates of the new model has widened, and now includes advocates in family and primary care medicine, psychiatry and other therapy fields, and the allied field of medical sociology.

These disciplines have developed over the past two decades and today constitute a countercurrent to the growing specialization and fragmentation of both medical thinking and medical care. Marked often by an allegiance to primary-care or family-centered medicine, the new trend has emphasized continuing and comprehensive care in contrast to episodic, compartmentalized, or fragmented care. Its broader model of disease fits its view of the broader world in which it moves, and the broader psychosocial task medical professionals are asked to fulfill. This new movement in health care has appealed to many levels of society: to those concerned with the escalating costs of medical care as well as those dedicated to a more intimate and enduring doctor-patient relationship which could continue the most compassionate aspects of medical tradition.

Melded into this new movement—though not without some contention—are two main groups of physicians: 1) the primary-care specialties of internal medicine, obstetrics-gynecology, and pediatrics; and 2) the newly resurgent field of family medicine. In some parts of the country, notably where the academic departments of the already-established specialties were weak, family practice has grown rapidly. In the more traditional centers, the primary-care movement has been led by the liberal and progressive wings of the primary-care specialties already in powerful positions. Much of the dispute has centered around the question of government funds and medical school teaching time.

In particular, the development of family medicine as a new discipline has offered the countercurrent trend an opportunity to change the look of American medicine. Instead of having 80% of physicians being specialists, this discipline holds the reverse to be more appropriate; further, family medicine is in a position to spearhead such a reorganization of medical care, taking on the associated questions of how care should be organized, payment schemes, the role of ancillary medical staff, office-hospital relations, and so on.

To date, however, the new field has not taken political or ideological leadership of medical change. In fact, it has often closely adhered to prevailing medical notions. Even when its practical activity has led it to deal with families as units of care, it has tended tó continue to view medicine along the perspective of the specialists—individuals, organ systems, etc.

In essence, actually, most of the basic biomedical views embodied in medical teaching and medical practice have yet to be examined critically at all.

Such is certainly the case with *diagnosis*.

The most recent works in the field have all started from the viewpoint that diagnosis is a brilliant act of reasoning in the clinician's mind. They have not, therefore, been able to guide physicians whose experience has advanced their perspective beyond a mechanistic mode.

A new approach, however, is slowly developing. Applying insights from general systems theory, it approaches medical problems in a systemic way, emphasizing both the *context* in which things occur and the *interrelationships* among the different parts of the phenomenon under scrutiny. This book attempts to apply such an approach to the keystone problem of diagnosis.

DIAGNOSIS AS A SOCIAL EVENT

Most discussions of diagnosis today focus on its being a masterful art, a process internal to the physician's mind, which combines scientific knowledge, clinical observation, and intuition. Physicians receive advice on how to recognize subtle signs of disease, are taught to memorize formulas and syndromes, and are warned not to "overlook" an illness. The brilliant clinician pursues illnesses whose existence can be objectively verified.

While few might contest the importance of organizing knowledge at the highest possible level, there is more to the problem of diagnosis than inductive and deductive thinking, for the creation of a diagnosis is a complicated social process. *Diagnosis, whatever else it may be, is essentially a social event.* It is a process whereby one person (the qualified expert) affixes a classification onto another person (the identified patient).

The process has several parts. In one sense, a diagnosis is a "working hypothesis" which will guide all subsequent treatment. This area is essentially epistemological and contains questions about the physician's skill and depth of knowledge, as well as considerations of "truth," "certainty," "probability," "proof," and so on. In another sense, a diagnosis is an agreed-upon, mutually-negotiated contract between people. Here, questions of process and context emerge. Finally, a diagnosis is a label whose consequences for the patient extend far beyond the medical realm, affecting especially the social and political spheres, with severe repercussions in a person's economic well-being as well.

The most helpful conceptual framework with which to understand this process derives from general systems theory, and has been popularly referred to as "systems thinking" or a "systems approach" (Ashby, 1956; Bateson, 1972; Laszlo, 1972; von Bertalanffy, 1968). Rather than examine illness in a strictly linear way, looking for cause-and-effect one-to-one relationships, systems thinking approaches the process emphasizing both the *context* in which things occur (the symptoms, the decision to see the doctor, the manner with which the complaints are offered up) and the *interrelationships* among the different factors involved (the timing of the illness, the interaction between the patient's complaints and the physician's workup, the role of stress in work and family life, the relationship between genetic predisposition and inciting events). A systemic approach does not abandon linear relationships if they are helpful in clarifying the patient's problems. But it does tend to emphasize the overall pattern and context in which the illness is situated.

When the phenomenon of reaching a diagnosis is explored from such a framework, three main aspects emerge:

1) *Diagnosis as knowledge.* This raises the question of diagnosis as fact vs. "working hypothesis." It looks at the degree of certainty or uncertainty in the diagnosis, and into the nature of illness itself, as well as the traditional notions of skill and training, and scientific method.
2) *Diagnosis as process.* This aspect considers contextual and broadly interactional aspects of the diagnostic process, as well as the eventual "social contract" arrived at.
3) *Diagnosis as a label.* This aspect looks at the social and political aspects of the diagnosis, as well as the medical or health consequences of being treated for that particular "illness" by the medical system.

Although many levels of systems are involved in making a diagnosis—from the molecular to the organ system, to the individual, the family, and the social surround—practically speaking, physicians are most likely to be dealing with the interaction among the individual patient, his or her family, and the medical world. The relationship between physician and patient can be seen as the "tip of the iceberg" which extends more deeply into both the family/social world in which the patient is embedded and the complex medical system at whose edge the physician may often be perched.

Diagnosis, far from being a simple mental event, thus represents social dialogue, social conflict, and social contracting.

INTEGRATING BIOMEDICAL AND PSYCHOSOCIAL FACTORS

But diagnosis is not confined to the interpersonal interaction in which it takes place. Our understanding of illness has widened to include a variety of etiological and precipitating factors: from pollutants in the air and environment to job-related hazards and carcinogens; from the effects of stress on an individual's cardiovascular system to the workings of frustration, anxiety, and loss on his or her immune system; and to the effects of family factors on the illnesses its members develop. What has been called the "psychosomatic premise"—that bodily events have emotional consequences and vice versa—has by now been so widely accepted that it is a part of our cultural heritage.

Diagnosticians thus no longer automatically look for the "single cause" of a given illness. They understand that illnesses occur in particular settings, that they are dealt with in different ways by different individuals and their families (and by different physicians), and that they are capable of affecting the world about them, and being affected by it. In addition, many issues usually in the purlieu of treatment or management can also be viewed as aspects of diagnostic medicine. (For example, if a chest pain responds to nitroglycerin, it is more likely to be angina than if it does not; if stomach cramps and dyspepsia respond to simple sedatives and anti-spasmodics, they are more likely due to an irritable stomach disorder than to an ulcer; if a headache responds to Cafergot but not to Fiorinal, it is more likely to be migraine than tension headache; and so on.)

The clinician's task then becomes weighing the factors which might contribute to the patient's distress or affect its treatment, and deciding which of them to pursue. Usually this means figuring out how to handle the relationship between physical and psychosocial issues.

Before going further along this line, though, we must acknowledge that most people initially go to their physician because of some *physical* malaise. They feel ill. They think something is wrong, somewhere, with their body. Perhaps their body is not functioning correctly. Perhaps something bad is happening to it. Patients do not know, so they go to their doctor for an answer. The patient usually does not say, "Something is askew in my psychosocial milieu, so I'll go to the doctor and ask him about it." Not at all. They go with their complaints of belly pains, headaches, or "just plain feeling tired and dragged out." If the physician fails to respond to their initial concerns, they will stop being his patients.

Physicians, *especially* those who apply a broader, systems perspective to diagnosis, must therefore respond to this basic concern. If they do not, they will ultimately lose access both to patients' physical and to their psychosocial ills.

In other words, medical care has to begin with a respect and appreciation for the patient's physical suffering and complaints. Physicians have to listen to their patients' announced complaints, physical or otherwise, and perform an examination which is appropriate to such presenting symptoms. I say this in the conviction that medicine may be (and should be) strongly affected by social science; however, its starting point has to be physicians' sensitivity to their patients' bodily distress.

After all, the expertise of physicians comes from the collective public conviction that they are adept at dealing with bodily ills: They can understand and heal them. Whatever understanding of psychosocial forces physicians achieve, they must—at least at this point in time in the U.S.—begin with the patient's own complaints, which are more often than not physical.

Having accepted this, though, physicians must then choose how far to go in exploring psychosocial issues. With all but the most simple, acute illnesses, the depth of insight they gain into the patient's life situation can deepen their grasp of "what is happening," thereby leading to a better diagnosis and making them better able to help the patient. Here is where conflict between the patient's view of what the doctor should be doing and the doctor's own view often breaks forth sharply.

While it is relatively easy to begin with the patient's announced physical problems, it may be difficult to continue doing only that, especially when the physician senses that the physical problems are rooted in a broader emotional context. Several factors are involved in this. First, both popular and professional understanding of the relationship between emotions and physical illness is very uneven. While some physicians have now learned a great deal about the unity between "mind" and "body," many have not. In addition, some patients have been so well schooled in the older medical model that they resist a more integrated view of medical care. They go along with the specialists' view that the best medical care is the most specialized—and also the most costly. This may lead to tension between a physician who senses that there is more to the patient's presenting problem than the patient is willing to allow and the patient who, with the support of other family members and even other physicians, may insist on pursuing a physical approach to his problem, even when the physician feels it is not appropriate to keep on doing so.

Second, the breakthroughs in current research around relations between emotions and physical illness—e.g., in psychoneuroimmunology—have not been well translated into popular terms. Thus, many patients who might support a more integrated concept have not obtained access to the information which would help them do it. Oddly enough, the conventional wisdom has always held that the mind affects the body, and vice versa; however, patients, even those who believe this, still expect their physicians to be experts in bodily distress and may feel it is inappropriate for them to wander from this focus.

A third problem involves the many patients with more than one illness. The elderly especially have a wide number of physical ailments, as well as much "functional" and situational distress—anxiety, worry, fear, guilt, and depression. The physician who would deal simultaneously with both their emotional and their physical needs must be quite skillful. In such a setting, physical concerns constantly emerge, often overshadowing the deeper emotional problems, and most physicians will be impelled to focus on the pressing biomedical problems and relegate emotions to second place.

A fourth difficulty involves the patients who have become virtual addicts to the medical model. They have learned it too well, and are now the chronic complainers, chronic patients, and chronic "doctor shoppers," strongly resisting anyone's efforts to integrate psychosocial and somatic considerations. They are unwilling to deal with their distress at an emotional, as well as physical, level and consequently become mired in what Huygen and Smits have called "somatic fixation" (1983).

Other difficulties rest on the current organization of medical care and the values it imparts. Patients feel that "you get what you pay for" and look towards hospital-based care and specialist care as the best. The ensuing fragmentation of services reinforces a fragmentation of understanding. While patients entrust their organ systems to different physicians, they often have no generalist who is able and willing to integrate their overall care. Fragmentation of care can lead to a spiraling of confusion. Specialists may disagree with one another. So may family members. Situations develop in which patients are trapped in a baffling matrix: The diagnosis is unclear; the treatment plan is unclear; different doctors and different family members each advocate a different solution, and so on.

Medicine today is a pluralistic system, and many points of view compete. The point of view which advocates an overall, integrated perspective is but one voice among the many.

Physicians who argue for the critical role of a systems-oriented medical generalist (family physician) must be able to help educate their patients, as well as cope with bias in other medical care providers, attitudes which would chop patients into a dozen organ systems, separate them from their families and social context, and offer them many simultaneous specialists, but not one trained generalist.

Many difficulties arise, of course, in trying to "listen" to the patient's physical complaints. It is often unclear just *what* is wrong, *why* it has gone wrong, and *how* it has happened. In addition, it is not always clear what all this *means* to the patient, and how the physician should interpret these complaints.

Physical complaints are not always simple to diagnose. There are, beyond the questions of focusing on the organ system responsible, questions of test reliability, diagnostic error, errors of interpretation by radiologists and pathologists, and honest differences of opinion. The facts, even when all put together neatly, may admit of more than one possibility, or they may be too confused to indicate any one disease. Finding an abnormality may not necessarily mean that the abnormality is the *cause* of the patient's distress. (For example, finding gallstones in a patient with abdominal pain may or may not provide an explanation of the pain.)

As we shall see, then, even when the physician acknowledges the patient's concern with his or her physical malaise, it may be difficult to come up with a satisfactory diagnostic explanation.

This, too, then is part of diagnosis. It leads to questions of how "broad" a diagnosis needs to be in order best to manage patients and their illness. How comprehensive an understanding will one need in order to manage the patient, the illness, and the concerned family? How comprehensive an understanding is needed to feel that one has "understood" the problem?

Such an exploration leads to questions of epidemiology and of epistemology, questions surrounding the role of family dynamics and family patterns, as well as even more sophisticated questions involving the biophysiology of the body's functioning, its relationship to humoral factors, and its linkage to genetic givens.

Physicians who, sensitively starting with their patients' announced complaints, try to unravel them to the best of their ability may find that this diagnostic effort carries them to new terrains. The reexamination of diagnosis, in short, is part of an overall examination of medical thought and practice. It must be seen as a component part of the effort to develop a better paradigm with which to approach matters of health and disease, and around which to organize the training and activity of physicians in the coming years.

Part I
Analysis

CHAPTER 1

Diagnosis: A Clinical Example

Aaron M, a 75-year-old widower, comes to the emergency room accompanied by his youngest daughter and her boyfriend. He is complaining of severe "pressures" in his chest, which have lasted for several days in spite of his having taken dozens of nitroglycerin pills. He is also weak and short of breath, and states he has "lost his appetite."

The emergency room physician has never seen Mr. M before. He checks his vital signs, takes a history from both the patient and his family, and carries out a physical examination, which is basically normal. He then orders blood tests and an EKG. The blood tests are normal. The EKG, while unchanged from previous tracings, nonetheless shows signs of damage to the heart muscle. Worried, the physician admits Mr. M to the hospital ICU with the tentative diagnosis of "crescendo angina" and calls in a cardiologist, Dr. V, to manage the case there.

By the time he reaches the ICU, Mr. M is agitated and confused. He is waving his arms around and shouting. The nurses note that he is mumbling to himself and giggling inappropriately, and he keeps asking for more nitroglycerin. The daughter, kept out of the ICU by hospital policy, appears frantic. She announces that she will not leave, but will keep a vigil by Mr. M's bedside until he is better. She also demands to know where the cardiologist is, and when she plans to see her father. The nurses order immediate blood gases, tell the daughter to try to calm down, and hook up an IV and a cardiac monitor. They are about to give

3

Mr. M a sedative when the daughter says he is "allergic" to all tranquilizers, and they should not give him anything without checking his
medical records first.

The cardiologist arrives and, after examining Mr. M, increases his anti-
angina medications. In her view, Mr. M is an elderly gentleman with
generalized arteriosclerosis, impaired blood flow to the brain, and dam-
aged coronary arteries. By his history, the patient has already experienced both a stroke and a heart attack; he has undergone surgical repair
for narrowing of the blood vessels to his head; and his pulses are di-
minished. Medical treatment is, therefore, intensified in order to stem
the cresting pains.

The family physician, who has known Mr. M for years (but who is
not permitted to manage patients in the ICU), knows that he has been
increasingly depressed since his wife died seven years ago. Thinking
about her, he often breaks down and cries. For several years, his youngest daughter had lived with him and taken care of him, but now she
has moved out, is living with a roommate, and is seriously dating her
current boyfriend, whom she plans to marry.

This change has coincided with Mr. M's growing increasingly confused. Unable to cook for himself, he has been eating irregularly, often
going to the local Jack-in-the-Box, where he has a hamburger, a soda,
and some french fries. He has also been complaining of chest pains more
frequently, which he treats with nitroglycerin. At times, when the pains
persist, he phones his daughter and tells her (apologetically) that he is
heading to the nearest emergency room, and asks her to meet him there.
She then drops whatever she is doing and calls her boyfriend; the two
of them rush to the hospital, usually just in time to see Mr. M being
admitted.

The daughter, Jennie, has become more and more worried. "We can't
just leave him alone," she has said to the family physician. "Maybe I
should get married, and then he could come and live with us." She is
also furious with her older sibs and half-sibs, feeling that the "whole
burden" for her father's care has come down on her.

The physician also recalls that Mr. M grows more disorganized each
time he is hospitalized. He confuses day with night. His speech rambles,
and he often giggles inappropriately. It seems as if his mind melts in
strange surroundings, and he often has to be restrained, much to his
family's consternation. Sedation only makes him more disorganized,
and he has developed wild and shrieking reactions to such medication
as Librium or Valium. If he is not tied down, however, he is likely to

be found wandering the hospital corridors, clad in two or three pairs of pants, looking for a phone.

To the family physician, Mr. M's appearance in the emergency room signals his increasing distress over his family situation. Of course, he has a number of sicknesses. But the drama of his repetitive presentation in the emergency room, with daughter and boyfriend in close attendance, points to an unravelling family problem as well as to a medical illness. The harmful consequences of this family problem appear to include exacerbating Mr. M's angina, as well as constantly disrupting several different people's lives, at rather considerable medical expense.

The hospital staff and specialists do not agree with this. They place Mr. M in the ICU, increase his medication, and deal with him as a "cardiac" case. The patient's family actually appears comfortable with this approach, and they seem to prefer discussing his medical problems rather than exploring their own response to his intractable complaining.

Thus, the medical problem expands to include conflicts at different levels: between the family physician and the specialist, between the office-based practice and the emergency room, between Mr. M and his daughter, between the daughter and the rest of the family, and between family members and the different physicians involved. What is the diagnosis?

CHAPTER 2

The Traditional View of Diagnosis: Medical Genius at Work

For centuries, medicine has viewed diagnosis as a process in the physician's mind. This process, akin to the artist's or writer's creative act, blends the physician's clinical observation and judgment with his or her knowledge of different disease entities, capacity to reason both inductively and deductively, and intuition. According to this view, the illness exists "out there," as a fact. The physician gathers necessary data—through taking a history, examining the patient, obtaining X-rays and other laboratory procedures—and then, reflecting on the different diagnostic possibilities, reaches a conclusion about the particular disease the patient is suffering.

Diagnosticians' skill is usually gauged by noting how often their diagnoses jibe with objective reality. Are they usually right or wrong? After all, there can be no middle ground. Since treatment must fit the presumed diagnosis, physicians whose diagnoses are most frequently correct will be most likely to cure their patients, and are therefore the best clinicians.

According to this view, the clinician is always trying to visualize the *disease*. The patient frequently seems to be in the way. As Ransom (1982) has observed, "The modern biomedical model still views the patient as a dirty window through which the physician must peer to 'see' the disease." Such a view goes along with physicians' traditional conduct,

6

placing themselves on a pedestal as the authority, and insisting that patients trust them and carefully follow their instructions. In recent years, this stance has encountered strong resistance and criticism from consumer groups and from patients who feel they have a right to a more symmetrical relationship. Yet, it remains the prevalent attitude of practicing physicians, who cite the tremendous advances of modern medicine in the past 150 years as justification.

ENGLE AND DAVIS

An excellent and comprehensive presentation of the traditional view is found in Engle and Davis's article "Medical diagnosis: present, past, and future," which appeared in the *Archives of Internal Medicine* (1963). Erudite and sophisticated, this review provides a well-reasoned brief for the biomedical view of diagnosis.

The authors begin by commenting:

> Diagnosis is such an established part of medical practice that few physicians consider whether there is general agreement about what is meant by the term diagnosis; whether diagnosis is an art, a science, or both; whether diagnosis is an essential prerequisite to medical management; and even whether diagnoses are clearly defined disease entities. (p. 512)

They then note the importance both physicians and lay people place on diagnosis, commenting that both experience "relief" and "satisfaction" when a diagnosis is reached. However, even though diagnosis so significantly decreases anxiety, one should not forget that "diagnosis . . . is based on concepts of disease which have many limitations."

The authors then define diagnosis as:

> the art, science, or act of recognizing disease from signs, symptoms, or laboratory data. It also signifies the decision reached. (p. 513)

From this essentially physician-centered view, they then move to consider such other categories linked to diagnosis, as *nosology, classification,* and *nomenclature.* They have no doubt that diseases do in fact objectively exist. Yet, hedgingly, they raise the question, "Does one diagnose a patient or a disease?" and respond that "One diagnoses the disease in a patient."

They then discuss the "process" of diagnosis, by which they mean the *mental process* the physician follows to arrive at a diagnosis, the act of scientific reasoning, intuition, or "kind of creative effort." They view this "process" as entirely internal.

Next they consider diagnosis as "the decision reached." This can be considered narrowly and precisely, as in Sydenham's (1858) original concept that disease entities are discrete species, like the species in biology. Or it can be viewed more broadly, as Clark-Kennedy's position that a diagnosis should be "a brief descriptive statement of [the] patient . . . the pathological process or processes . . . and the structural changes and functional disturbances." (The latter statement reflects centuries of gradual rarefaction and development of the concept of disease, whose history is summed up in a later section of the Engle and Davis paper.)

All of this focuses on the physician's attempt to probe and define the aberrant disease process. The authors never consider the physician's interaction with the patient.

Engle and Davis then move to consider the purposes of diagnosis. They identify three: 1) the naming and classification of disease; 2) the reinforcement of an entire "set of attributes and theory . . . which constitute the science of medicine"; and 3) the stimulation of further investigation. Essentially, this means that each diagnosis serves to reinforce the medical model which has created it.

They then discuss the lack of a "unified concept of disease," which leads to "limitations" in diagnosis. Not all physicians approach an illness in the same way; not all diseases have universally accepted definitions; some diseases have changeable characteristics. Because of these presently unavoidable limitations, the authors propose a gamut of five "orders of certainty" with which any particular diagnosis can be made.

This schema deals, however, only with physical illnesses. It organizes illnesses according to a level of certainty with which they can be diagnosed. The gamut depends on whether one can isolate the "causative agent" of the disease; whether the presentation of the disease is typical or varies from patient to patient; and whether the pathological reactions involved in the disease are understood. Based on these criteria, a spectrum of certainty is drawn out, from broken bones, harelip, burns, and frostbite (Level 1), to pneumonia and strep throat (Level 2), to cirrhosis, peptic ulcer, and essential hypertension (Level 3), to cancers and osteoarthritis (Level 4), to lupus, sarcoidosis, and Loeffler's syndrome (Level 5).

This discussion of certainty is very frustrating. To begin with, it is arbitrary and inexact. In addition, it ignores any "functional" illness. Its overall point is quite true, however: Some diseases are *obvious*, even to the uncultured eye. As a disease process becomes more and more difficult to figure out, the level of certainty for its diagnosis falls. This explains the persistent disagreement among physicians, even regarding physical illnesses. (As we will see later, questions of certainty can become exceedingly complicated, especially when applied to some of the most common illnesses and to the mix between emotional and physical factors.)

Such a view of diagnosis is echoed in virtually all medical textbooks, most of which fail to devote more than a few lines to the concept. The traditional view works best when it comes to obvious diseases which can be diagnosed by the man in the street ("Doc, I think she's got a broken leg"), when the illness is simple, the causative agent single and clear, and the disease process evident to the five human senses. Thus, a fractured tibia, a draining boil, and large bleeding hemorrhoids are all fairly simple to diagnose, with a high level of certainty. (There may, of course, be a dispute over the best treatment, but this is not the issue being discussed here.)

The farther afield one moves from strict "linear" relationships—when one tries to unravel the cause of hypertension, for example, or of an "irritable bowel syndrome," or of vague and unsettling "chest pains"—the harder this traditional notion of diagnosis becomes, and the greater is the acknowledged degree of *un*certainty.

Some hold that such uncertainty stems only from our lack of detailed knowledge. Applying the mechanistic world model (Pepper, 1942) to illness, they hold that all processes could be explored and understood—if only we had the tools necessary to the task. Thus, to clarify the mystery of irritable bowel syndrome versus some other diagnosis, they would be pleased by the development of newer, more sophisticated tests—CT-scans, ERCP, biopsy, colonoscopy. Uncertainty, the mechanists hold, does not exist "out there," but "in here"—in the limitations of our own scientific approach. They hold that uncertainty essentially stems from ignorance. A contrasting approach will be discussed later, namely that uncertainty is part of the world "out there" and that medical diagnoses must be arranged on a "probabilistic" spectrum (Bursztajn et al., 1981).

Engle follows this first article with a second (1963a), tracing the concept of diagnosis from prehistoric times to the present, and then grappling with philosophical questions underlying diagnosis. His bent is towards a more sophisticated system of classification, and his analysis leads him to the medical use of computers. Indeed, his final article (1963b) is a strongly worded brief for the use of computer technology in solving problems of medical diagnosis.

FEINSTEIN

Another quite scholarly approach to diagnosis emerges in Feinstein's 1967 monograph, *Clinical Judgment*. Interestingly, Feinstein also pursues a strictly biomedical view of disease, and struggles with the varying presentations of different diseases: diseases which produce symptoms, and those which do not, and those which may and/or may not. Just as Engle's questions of how to handle the intricate mass of data lead him to computer application, Feinstein's interest in the overlapping sets which constitute a disease picture or syndrome leads him to an application of Boolean algebra.

Citing Claude Bernard, Feinstein begins by criticizing clinical medicine for getting immersed in the "why" of illness instead of pursuing the "how." This introduces a discussion of ways of organizing data, potential sources of error, and the fallacy of seeking out single causes rather than observing the overlapping and diverse presentations of disease states.

He criticizes diagnosis for relying on morbid anatomy, whose proof is often unavailable until after a patient has died (as in myocardial infarction), and points out that abnormal function is as much a disease process (perhaps more so) as abnormal structure. Furthermore, a single disease state may have very different presentations: primary cancer, locally metastatic cancer, widely disseminated cancer; cancer-producing symptoms, cancer-not-producing symptoms. The diagnosis usually given a patient's problem may obliterate the unique distinctions the patient presents.

Feinstein then discusses *taxonomy*. He argues that

> the main diagnostic taxonomy used by clinicians today depends on the concepts and nomenclature of morbid anatomy observed by pathologists . . . myocardial infarction, phlebothrombosis . . . multiple sclerosis . . . diverticulitis . . . Not a single one of these diagnostic terms represents an entity that is ever actually seen, heard, or touched in the ordinary bedside observations of a clinician. (Feinstein, 1967, p. 71)

Arguing that the clinician must diagnose "a host *and* an illness *and* a disease," he develops a lengthy historical and philosophical argument aimed at restoring the primacy of the clinician's observations to the notion of diagnosis. He does this by classifying two *approaches* to disease (empirical and hypothetical) and three *types of data* (clinical manifestations, anatomic manifestations, and etiologic inferences contained in theories). Thus, Sydenham typifies the empirical approach; Sylvius and the iatrochemists, the hypothetical one.

Finally, Feinstein traces the historical development of both morbid anatomy and physiology, and concludes that current diagnostic terms are out of date because they cling to a model of morphological abnormality, while the clinician deals with the complex picture of dysfunction, protean manifestations of any disease process, and so on. He concludes that medical taxonomy is inadequate; it offers no adequate terms for the interaction between host, disease process, and clinical symptoms produced.

> Human taxonomy provides a classification for designating a host who has a disease. Pathologic taxonomy provides a classification for designating (or diagnosing) the host's disease. There is no organized medical system, however, for classifying the illness that is the clinical interaction of host and disease. (p. 127)

From this frustrating point, Feinstein then moves to categorize the signs and symptoms of physical disease, the clinical attributes of symptoms and signs (iatrotropy, toponymy, and chronometry); then, following the schema which he constructs, he develops a mathematical approach to different clinical diseases. The intricacies of his approach are beyond the realm of this book, as is his use of Venn diagrams and Boolean intersecting sets. (The interested reader will find his book a fascinating and rewarding expedition into the "hard" scientific organization of data about the known physical diseases.) My point is that, having stated the problem quite clearly, he then moves away from any psychosomatic terrain and works only to update the 19th century notion of disease. He tries to reform the notion of physical disease while avoiding any emotionally linked problems.

The parabola of his thought veers towards a systemic approach, only to recede from it. Feinstein leaves a feeling of being overwhelmed by the *data* of disease, which must all be scientifically organized to give meaning. But, ironically and unfortunately, the further his argument goes, the further afield it moves from clinical experience. His is a masterful work, rich in its grasp of probability and statistical variation—but lacking an entry to the affective and experiential life of the "host."

SUMMARY

Aside from these two scientific discussions of diagnosis, there has been little substantial investigation of the phenomenon. Most textbooks devote a paragraph or two to the topic, talking primarily about the clinician's skill. Medical students are trained in the detective-story Clinical-Pathological-Conference (CPC), in which an astute clinician tries to make a diagnosis from the available data, and then is complemented by the pathologist, who has found out "the" right answer for everyone. What Feinstein bemoans—the lack of a real nosology to fit the clinician's desire for an all-embracing description—is yet to be confronted by the medical school academics.

Thus, the traditional notion constantly falls short of what is needed; but, as if in some fairyland, "no one seems to notice." Physicians mechanically fall back on the available diagnostic terms, apparently not even noting that some of them bear little resemblance to the clinical pictures presented.

The traditional notion, which has succeeded so well with infectious illnesses and other "obvious" medical problems and emergencies, founders badly when it comes to the wide range of family practice problems, patients with vague complaints and mixed (psychosomatic, stress-related) illnesses. The traditional notion has trouble explaining differences of host resistance or disease "expression." And it has difficulty dealing with even simple diseases whose full picture involves complex relationships between environmental, immunological, epidemiological, infectious, and psychological factors (such as rheumatoid arthritis, bronchial asthma, or atopic eczema). While the model works well when one particular cause seems mainly responsible, it stumbles at interrelated causative factors.

For example, if a patient visits the physician complaining of epigastric pain, the traditional model of diagnosis can readily proceed to deal with possible physical causes—hiatus hernia, peptic ulcer, gallstones, gastroenteritis. If the workup shows one of these causes, there is an answer. If the workup is negative, the physician can hold to the undocumented gastroenteritis—watching its clinical course closely—and can be satisfied if the problem clears. If the problem persists, perhaps a diagnosis may be made of "subacute" this or that, or the physician may feel that the X-ray studies are wrong, and the patient does indeed have gallstones, or that the patient suffers from "diverticulosis" (a wastebasket diagnosis in this case), or perhaps from a psychosomatic disorder, such as "irritable bowel syndrome." How the physician actually *decides* probably has more to do with his or her particular bias than with any subsequently found data. The more biomedically oriented may go so far as further, more elaborate tests—endoscopy, exam of the stool, small bowel biopsy—only to throw up their hands if everything is "negative." (The biomedically oriented must find disease or they are lost—they are like the Cookie Monster in an orange grove, desperate for familiar food.)

Of course, even finding a "peptic ulcer" does not end the questioning. What has brought this ulcer into existence? Is it secretion of acid? Which cells have done this? Is it a failure of regulation, of inhibition, of facilitation, of excitation. . . ? What is the role of biological factors? Heredity? How much are environmental factors involved, like smoking, alcoholic intake, coffee drinking? And, of course, how are these latter related to cultural patterns, work habits, and stress? Is alcoholic intake being used to kill the pain, to avoid relationships, to be "one of the boys," to get high? Is there a family pattern of such behavior, and of ulcers? The questions go on *ad infinitum*. How can the simple biomedical model answer them?

The mind/body dichotomy lurks as a dilemma throughout biomedicine, for its model of disease can only be physical, somatic. The contributions of psychological factors, unless somehow titratable in biochemical or physiological terms (free fatty acid level, galvanic skin response) are *outside* the discussable, verifiable universe. They are delegated to the specialist in that world, the psychiatrist or psychologist, who can more properly deal with those vague phenomena—with the result that now, as in Descartes' time, the realm of the mind and the realm of the body remain distinct, separate, and barely related coeval worlds, each with its own physicians to tend the infirm.

For these and other reasons, then, the traditional notions of diagnosis (and disease) merit strong reexamination, in order to bring them up more in line with our experience and need.

CHAPTER 3

Critiques of the Traditional View

Critiques of the biomedical view have come from both outside and inside of medicine.

OUTSIDE OF MEDICINE

A number of biologists and philosophers of science have examined the 19th century medical model and found it inadequate to explain natural phenomena. Foremost among them is Rene Dubos, Nobel Prize laureate, whose monograph, *The Mirage of Health* (1979), challenges many assumptions held by physicians today and widely taught in medical schools.

Dubos begins his book by acknowledging people's hopes for cure from disease, and for a healthy world. But this wish, he notes, is at odds with the facts of life. For:

> Life is an adventure in a world where nothing is static; where unpredictable and ill-understood events constitute dangers that must be overcome, often blindly and at great cost; where man himself, like the sorcerer's apprentice, has set in motion forces that are potentially destructive and may someday escape his control. . . . Complete and lasting freedom from disease is but a dream remembered from imaginings of a Garden of Eden designed for the welfare of man. (pp. 1-2)

14

He then traces the notions of health and disease that reigned prior to the triumph of the specific etiology of disease. For centuries, people believed that sickness represented an imbalance of forces between sick people and their environment, a "lack of harmony," as it were. Not only was this compatible with the exploration of social and environmental factors affecting disease—a tendency which was growing in the first part of the 19th century—but it was also consistent with folk wisdom throughout the ages and with the contemporary movement towards "whole person" medicine.

The great biological discoveries of the 19th century changed all this. By finding the specific agents responsible for anthrax, tuberculosis, syphilis, and so on, medicine adopted a new theory: the doctrine of the "specific etiology of disease." This doctrine held that every disease had a single cause, and that once the cause was determined specific therapy could be directed at it. This belief has reigned in medicine for the past hundred years and is still dominant today.

Dubos, however, points out that the doctrine of specific etiology fails to grapple successfully with many of the afflictions that plague people today:

> Unquestionably the doctrine of specific etiology has been the most constructive force in medical research for almost a century, and the theoretical and practical achievements to which it has led constitute the bulk of modern medicine. Yet few are the cases in which it has provided a complete account of the causation of disease. Despite frantic efforts, the causes of cancer, of arteriosclerosis, of mental disorders, and of the other great medical problems of our time remain undiscovered. . . . In reality, search for *the* cause may be a hopeless pursuit because most disease states are the indirect outcome of a constellation of circumstances rather than the direct result of single determinant factors. (p. 102)

In fact, the model forged during the last century fails even to explain infectious illnesses. Dubos notes that almost everyone in the room when Koch read his epoch-making paper in 1882 had at some time been infected with tubercle bacilli. Yet only a small percentage of those affected had developed clinical disease. Similarly, Pettenkoffer and Metchnikoff "drank tumblerfuls of cultures isolated from fatal cases of cholera"; yet, although enormous quantities of cholera bacteria could be found in their stool, the experimenters suffered little more than mild diarrhea. Why was this? How could the theory of specific etiology explain such discrepant findings? Clearly, more was involved than simple exposure to the specific organism.

Such questions arise again and again in clinical medicine. An entire day-care classroom is exposed to strep throat; yet only some of the children develop the illness. An epidemic of gastroenteritis sweeps a factory; yet some workers fall ill and others do not. Beside the "offending organism," matters of host resistance and host susceptibility appear to be involved.

Nor is it a question only of the interaction between host and invading organism. The advances in reducing tuberculosis came more from the reforms in widespread sanitation and industrial hygiene than from particular antibiotics. In fact, the incidence of tuberculosis had begun to fall drastically *far before* the discovery of antibiotic therapy. Thus, there is interaction with the environment in which both host and organism live, an environment which combines natural and manmade factors.

The complexity of this basically systemic approach goes far beyond the doctrine of specific etiology.

Another major assault on the medical model of illness has come from relentless—but little disseminated—work in the allied field of medical sociology. From the initial incisive work of Talcott Parsons (1951) to the recent analysis of such writers as Freidson (1970), Zola (1966, 1983), Fox (1977), and Mishler et al. (1981), medical sociologists have applied their skills at studying the intricacies of the medical encounter and dissecting the medical profession as a social subsystem to create a cogent critique of the medical model of illness and the practice based upon it.

Foremost among current schools of sociological thought is the trend of social constructivism. This school argues that reality is fabricated through human action, that "the world as a *meaningful reality* is constructed through human interpretative activity" (Mishler et al., 1981). Mishler discusses the "social construction" of illness in a chapter whose outlook is similar to the one pursued in this volume. To a constructivist, he notes, "health, illness, and medical care are social facts." Behavior is looked upon differently by different classes, cultures, and subcultural groups—what appears "sick" to some people may be "normal" or "healthy" to others.

Rather than seeing illness as some fixed biomedical *given*, the constructivists view it as something worked out between people, between patients and their peers, or between patients and their doctors. People work at creating illness, developing it into a social entity. The discussion thus leads directly to an exploration of the *context* of disease, the patient's *attributions* of illness, *illness behavior*, and the political uses of the stamp of illness. (Mishler's examples are diabetes, hyperactivity, mental retardation, alcoholism, and blindness.)

At one pole, the constructivists' critique of the medical model blends into Illich's critique of the "medicalization of life" (1976). That is, physicians have the ability to create illness simply by pronouncing its name. One can even make a diagnosis these days of "no pathology" or "well baby visit," of "pain" or even of "rule out peptic ulcer." Categories exist to describe everything, and everything winds up being included in the medical world. Each discipline tends to view all others as "part" of itself, and medicine is no exception. The tendency is to see all of human experience as some kind of disease or non-disease process, and to make the physician, therefore, the final authority on politics, morality, suffering, ethics, sin, and merit . . . as well as on illness and its treatment. Such is the tendency Illich attacks. And the constructivists echo his critique.

At the other pole, the constructivists fall into a cynical pragmatism, asserting that things are simply what those in power name them—an approach which can claim more than a grain of truth.

Mishler's comments echo Freidson, who devoted one hundred pages in his major work (1970) to "the social construction of illness," arguing that physicians, by virtue of their social role, create illness as a social state: "Medicine creates the social possibilities for acting sick." Freidson is concerned with the labeling and subsequent management of what comes to be socially accepted as "sick."

This analysis may come as a shock and a surprise to physicians who have by and large convinced themselves that they are hard at work "discovering" the patient's illness. Freidson recognizes that the physician's diagnosis defines the situation and is accepted as correct by all those people concerned with the illness. The medical world *is* as the physicians say it is, regardless of any other "reality" going on in the patients' minds or bodies. Though this approach is not a complete picture of diagnosis either, it certainly adds a spicy ingredient which had been missing from the physicians' own descriptions of the phenomenon.

Critiques of the medical model have also come from "systems thinkers" in allied fields, especially from the family-oriented therapists who happen to have dealt with issues surrounding illness and how families grapple with them. Some of this criticism will emerge in later chapters.

WITHIN MEDICINE

As medicine has become more sophisticated in its outlook and especially in its technology, some criticism from within the field has been directed at the biomedical model of disease. The proliferation of elegant, carefully focused research activity, while leading to greater specialization on the one hand, has also unveiled the vast complexity involved in the disease process, thus making 19th-century causal notions seem crude and out of date. This has led to two trends: 1) the reformers, who cling to a basically physical notion of illness, and who are concerned (like Feinstein) with bringing it up to date, making it mathematically advanced, etc.; and 2) the proponents of an essentially new paradigm, who want to expand the notions of illness and its diagnosis to include broader psychosocial and other systemic issues. Pressures for change have also come from colleagues in the behavioral sciences who have been working closely with physicians in family medicine and other interdisciplinary programs, and who have been repelled by the old-line notion of diagnosis because it neglects family and psychological process.

Researchers into the nature of the stress response have deepened the earlier notions of psychosomatic illness (cf. Ader, 1981). Immunologists (Locke, 1982) have discovered much about the factors affecting host susceptibility and host resistance, as they study the effects of stress on the immune system. When such biophysiological data are combined with subjects' diary information about the stresses they are experiencing, the tools for investigating the interplay between psychosocial stresses and the body's physiological functioning have come together.

For years, general practitioners and other astute primary care providers have noted how illness "runs in families" (Kellner, 1963), have drawn up family patterns of illness (Peachey, 1963), and have noted variations in susceptibility to illness depending on different life stresses (Parkes, 1964). They have documented, for example, the devastating effects of losing one's spouse on one's susceptibility to disease (Rees and Lutkins, 1967), and have examined the effect on the rest of the family of one member's being ill (Klein et al., 1968; Widmer et al., 1980).

The accumulated weight of this work has demolished the notion of "one illness—one cause." Instead, a perspective has emerged which incorporates many interlocking factors. The best expression of this approach probably appears in the work of George Engel, whose "biopsychosocial" model of illness (1980) represents an attempt at forming a new paradigm in medicine, one which can assimilate the growing amount of relevant data about an entire disease process as it unfolds in a social surround.

Engel sees the natural world as a continuum of systems which interact at different levels. He holds to a view of the hierarchy of both natural and social worlds, from the smallest subatomic particles to atoms, molecules, proteins, small one-celled organisms, more complicated organisms, and so on, all the way to levels of individuals, couples, families, communities, and higher forms of social organization (see Figure 1). Any individual patient can be understood to participate in such a hierarchy of systems, and—in fact—to participate in a multiplicity of hierarchies. Such a concept dovetails into the familiar notion of having multiple roles ("I am a son, a father, a brother, a husband, a worker, a colleague, a tennis player, a friend. . . .") and of belonging to a number of different, distinct social groupings.

While such a gamut of systems is obvious, practically speaking, it has not been recognized by the medical world, for which its implications are staggering. Medical practice has mostly concerned itself with this or that abnormality going on at the organ or organ system level, occasionally (by the researchers) at the cellular or hormonal level, and (rarely) at the level of the patient as a "whole person." Opening up its perspective so that it includes interaction at various social and psychological levels goes beyond "reforming" the medical model: It substitutes a different, broader perspective which can embrace and utilize the traditional medical model but, at the same time, surpass it. It is akin to the shift from two to three dimensions as portrayed in the mathematical classic *Flatland* (Abbott, 1868).

Earlier views of the mind/body harmony have also been resurrected, as the critique of the medical model has gained force. The early psychosomatic thinkers struggled mightily to grasp the links between the emotions and bodily pathological processes. Was there organ specificity, they wanted to know. Did a particular personality type hold for each different illness? Did stress attack the "weakest link" in the body's different organ systems? Or was illness a more global response to the experience of loss? Questions went further. If the experience of loss was critical, did the loss have to be *actual*, or could a perceived loss do as well? Thus, investigators considered the stressful effects of the death of a spouse, the alienation of affection as manifested by divorce or marital stress, the anticipated loss of a job or a parent, the loss of self-esteem through perceived failures or frustrations, and so on.

Such questions, first asked in the early 1900s by those associated with the psychoanalytic movement, have reappeared, and are being asked again. This time, though, they can be asked with a higher degree of sophistication and with a greater sense of the hard epidemiological data that might be necessary to answer them. It is as if the process of knowl-

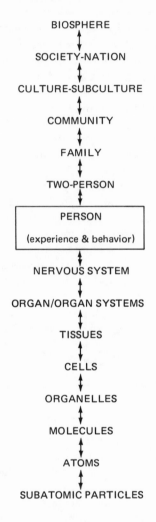

SYSTEMS HIERARCHY

(LEVELS OF ORGANIZATION)

BIOSPHERE
↕
SOCIETY-NATION
↕
CULTURE-SUBCULTURE
↕
COMMUNITY
↕
FAMILY
↕
TWO-PERSON
↕
PERSON
(experience & behavior)
↕
NERVOUS SYSTEM
↕
ORGAN/ORGAN SYSTEMS
↕
TISSUES
↕
CELLS
↕
ORGANELLES
↕
MOLECULES
↕
ATOMS
↕
SUBATOMIC PARTICLES

Figure 1. Hierarchy of natural systems (from Engel, 1980*).

edge is a spiral, with the same points being probed, only at higher or deeper levels (Figure 2).

In addition, it has long been clear that many patients' complaints do not fit into the known medical illnesses. Nor are they "new," undiscovered diseases. Especially in general or family practice, this has long been known, and is a source of steady frustration among practitioners trying to "manage" patients whose illnesses are not well understood, but are perceived to be related to a good deal of the daily stress they are experiencing.

Many patterns of patients' complaints are thus somatic expressions of anxiety, fear, and depression. Diagnoses which turn these into "functional" disorders may aid the practitioner by ascribing a context and

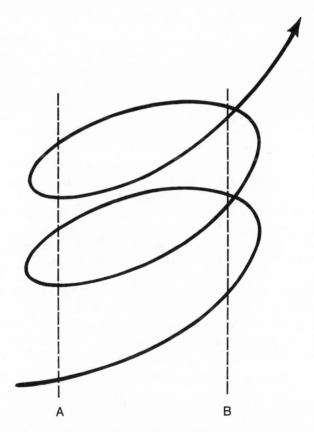

A   B

Figure 2. Spiral of knowledge.

influence to the symptoms, but they often do not help treat the patient, who hears the physician saying that "it's all in your head." And yet a wide range of the most common problems, comprising anywhere from 25-75% of a busy practitioner's day, fall into this category. The medical terms for them are legion: irritable bowel syndrome, angioneurotic edema, irritable stomach, neurodermatitis, chest wall pain, chronic pain syndrome, functional abdominal pain, psychophysiological gastrointestinal (or respiratory, or dermatological) reaction, tension headache, atypical migraine, and so on. The busy practitioner encounters these problems repeatedly in the course of a week's work, and yet there are few instructions on how to view these problems, how to explain them to patients, how to treat them, and how to study them in a scientific way.

The range of such symptoms can extend anywhere from the mildly disturbing and unsettling to the truly cataclysmic. Yet many patients who experience such symptoms (palpitations, fatigue, sighing, anorexia, heaviness, insomnia, listlessness, generalized achiness) reject any explanation which sounds the least bit psychological. "It's something *real*," they insist. "It's not my imagination. Are you saying that I'm nuts?"

As family medicine emerges as a legitimate field, one wing of the discipline has become increasingly concerned with psychosocial factors in illness, as well as with the interrelationship of illness and family process. After all, if the family is the "basic unit of medical care" (Schmidt, 1978), then the family physician has to be open to much more input about family dynamics, family emotional life, the stages of family growth, the different kinds of family stress, and so on. This is in direct challenge to the physician's remaining a skilled technician, an "expert" among lay people, a specialist. It forces physicians out of the groove into which the medical model and most of their training have thrust them, and encourages them to approach their patients with a broader view.

To date, however, such a "new physician" has often lacked the theoretical perspective which is needed to handle this task. The systems approach described in this book is intended to provide such a perspective, and to make the practitioner's life and work both more intelligible and more rewarding.

CHAPTER 4

Context for Diagnosis: The Meeting of Two Vast Systems

Physicians and patients do not exist in a vacuum. Neither are free, independent beings. Both belong to large, complicated, and often intersecting systems whose relationship to one another is constantly changing. These are the *family system* to which the patient belongs and the *medical system* to which the physician belongs. The relationship between the two can be expressed visually as two spheres, perpetually in motion, which are capable of engaging one another in any number of ways (Figure 3).

Whatever goes on between physician and patient happens in the context of these two systems. The relationship extends to involve large numbers of people who are linked to the patient and physician in different directions. At any given moment, the illness being diagnosed by the physician is being actively discussed by many other people within both of these intersecting systems, all of whom have some idea about what is "really" going on, who the real patient is, what problem is being manifested, and how it should be treated.

Although many levels of systems are involved in making a diagnosis—from the molecular level to the level of the organ system, to the individual, and to his or her social context—the levels which usually most concern the practicing physician are those of the individual and the family. Thus, we will focus here on the interaction between patient, physician, and family. The relationship between patient and physician can be seen as the "tip of the iceberg," extending more deeply into the social and familial contexts in which the patient is embedded and into the complex system which provides medical care, at whose edge the physician is often perched.

To understand the significance of this interaction, we must first explore what a "systems approach" is, beginning with the characteristics of a system.

SYSTEMS THEORY AND A SYSTEMS APPROACH

Systems theory has developed in the past 30 years as a way of understanding the complex, delicate organization of the world in which we live. It received a spur from the work with cybernetics and computers that began during World War II and expanded rapidly thereafter. It is a theory capable of dealing with a wide diversity of natural and social phenomena, from the very small to the very large, from human experience to the cold, impersonal objects of the micro- and macro-cosmos.

A system is a set of objects together with relationships between the objects and between their attributes (Hall and Fagen, 1978). Objects are another term for the parts of the system. Attributes are the properties of objects.

INTERACTION OF SYSTEMS

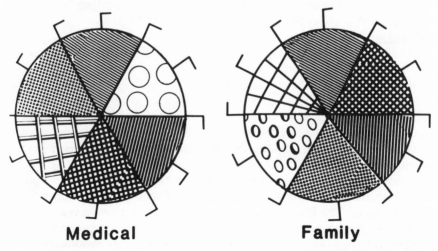

Medical   **Family**

Figure 3. Interaction of systems: Family system and medical system.

Relationships "tie the system together" and involve the parts in mutual interaction.

Systems can be static or dynamic, open or closed. *An open system exchanges materials, energy, or information with its environment.* It is thus capable of maintaining itself in spite of external stress, and is capable of change. Many natural systems are *adaptive*: They can react favorably to their milieux in order to endure and persevere. Many natural systems also have *feedback*, a property which permits self-regulation of activity in response to a variety of changes (such as a heater with a thermostat, or a human thyroid gland).

Systems are marked by certain characteristics:

1) The whole is greater than the sum of its parts. (A person is more than the sum of his or her different organ systems.)
2) Whatever affects the system as a whole affects each part. (Think of all the side effects any given medication, aimed at one particular problem, can arouse in a patient.)
3) Any change in one part affects the other parts and the system as a whole. (Any illness affects the whole patient; any illness in a family member affects the people he or she lives with.)

According to Beavers (1982), four basic assumptions mark a systems orientation:

1) An individual needs a group, a human system, for identity and satisfaction.
2) Causes and effects are interchangeable.
3) Human behavior is the result of many variables, rather than one "cause"; simplistic solutions are therefore questioned.
4) Human beings are limited and finite. No one is absolutely helpless or absolutely powerful in a relationship.

The quality of *wholeness* means that the system behaves as a whole, or "coherently" (Dell, 1982). The parts can only be understood in the context of the whole. The quality of *independence* refers to the degree of autonomy each part possesses within the whole.

Finally, natural systems form both a hierarchy and a continuum (Figures 1 and 4). The hierarchy of systems means that any given system may at the same time be a member of a larger system. The thyroid gland, for example, is a system in its own right, comprising its various cellular, structural, and functional properties. But it is, at the same time, a part of the endocrine system as a whole. And the endocrine system is but one organ system in the body as a whole. And so on. The continuum of systems expresses the increasing complexity of organization of natural and social systems, from the smallest cellular level to the aggregations of nations and peoples on this planet.

For further information on general systems theory, the interested reader is referred to the works of Buckley (1968), von Bertalanffy (1968), Ashby (1956), Laszlo (1972), and Hoffman (1981) cited in the bibliography.

In a systems perspective, emphasis focuses on the *interrelationships* among the parts, on the "glue" that holds the system together. Since living systems are dynamic entities, always coping with stress and

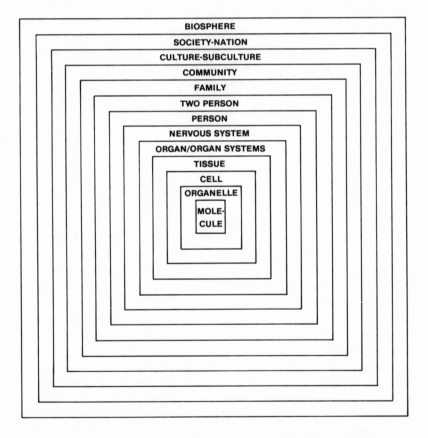

Figure 4. Continuum of natural systems (after Engel, 1980).

change, the interrelationships among their parts demonstrate what the system really does. A systems perspective looks at "process" and characterizes the communications and other transactions that occur between members.

Emphasis is also put on how systems handle change. Some living systems become *transformed* over time: An acorn becomes an oak; the baby becomes an adult. A tiny town grows into a city, then becomes a "ghost town" when its reason for growth recedes. An infection expands into an epidemic. An illness gives way to cure. A momentary worry develops into an all-involving obsession. This constant give-and-take between pressures for change (morphogenesis) and pressure for sameness (homeostasis) represents the dialectics of systems.

Systems thinking brings other changes into perspective, too. It focuses on context, looking to view and appreciate phenomena (behavior) in an all-sided, rather than a partial, way. Often this means investigating the social field in which behavior occurs, searching for its divers meanings and significance.

Such a view undercuts notions of simple causality and looks instead at *what* happens, rather than trying to figure out *why*. The tendency to go after the "how" rather than the "why" links it, scientifically, to the work of Claude Bernard, who, in his famous work, *The Introduction to the Study of Experimental Medicine* (1957), comments:

> The nature of our mind leads us to seek the essence or the *why* of things . . . (but) experience soon teaches us that we cannot get beyond the *how*. (p. 80)

A systemic perspective leads to describing patterns of recurrent behavior and sequences of interaction, rather than prolonged worry about which particular piece of behavior "comes first" or "causes" the others. This view has appealed to family therapists, for example, who enjoin the family not to cast blame on one particular member (the person who wickedly and maliciously "starts the arguments"), but rather to look at the patterns of behavior which surround and characterize family fights.

Such notions of causality have been dubbed "circular," as opposed to "linear." The implication is that systemic processes have no beginning and no end, but continue to evolve through time, showing patterns of one kind or another at different stages. Circular causality frees members from being to "blame" and is thus often therapeutic in psychotherapy. It can also be carried to an absurd extreme by dogmatic insistence—do the victim and the executioner form such a "system," the wife-beater and the beaten wife, the murderer and the sleeping victim?—thus losing sight of both common sense and the political content of people's acts. Still, compared to the "linear" thinking of the biomedical model, the move to circular thinking has to be seen as a liberating experience, opening up new possibilities and focusing on levels which were experienced before but never assessed.

From this viewpoint, several conclusions follow. To understand malfunction in any living system—illness, for example—one needs to grasp the system as a whole, not just one aspect. Disease, von Bertalanffy comments, "is the life process regulating toward normalcy after disturbance, owing to the equifinality of biological systems and with the assistance of the physician" (1968). (Equifinality refers to the fact that an open system may attain a time-independent state, independent of initial conditions and determined only by the system parameters.)

Homeostasis, about which much argument has occurred recently in family therapy, is attained only through great effort, for the world is constantly changing, and all living things are constantly being pressured to change with it. A dialectic world-view naturally follows, with conflict between forces of change and tendencies toward stability.

This begins to redefine causality, paving the way for notions of probability and uncertainty. It undermines the traditional notion of certainty, so dear to the doctrine of specific etiology and the "magic bullet" school of therapeutics, and makes the medical decision-making process much more complex. Such a change has, in fact, been occurring in recent years as witnessed by several volumes professing to aid the layman and physician in making decisions of a difficult moral or medical nature, whose consequences must be considered by a mathematics of probability (Bursztajn et al., 1981).

Although the hierarchy of systems can relate to factors quite large (the ecosphere's relation to physical illness), in actual practice the physician deals mostly with the family system and its relation to the medical system.

THE FAMILY SYSTEM

The patient belongs to the family system, a social unit itself in evolution. At present, all of us can boast of having been born into and raised by families of one form or another, and we usually have the tendency to recreate our families as we move through life. Criticisms of the 1960s notwithstanding, the family continues to exist and evolve, and is—for almost all of us—the main social unit to which we belong.

Medalie defines the family (1982) as:

> a group of intimate associates linked by blood, marriage, adoptive or fictive kin ties, who have mutual or common interests and activities, and who interact with each other for emotional, financial, and/or social support.

To this, we might add only that the family often has a common past and anticipates a common future.

The family is often focused around the household—people who live together—but important family members may live hundreds of miles away and still exert a powerful influence on family life. Even deceased family members may exercise a strong influence on subsequent generations, and may be instrumental in setting up family myths and legends, which not only are remembered over the years and passed down from generation to generation, but also have the power to become translated into fact, an example of how ideas transform reality. While the workings of this process are obscure, the fact that it does indeed operate this way is seen in countless numbers of alcoholic families, where third and fourth generation alcoholics can trace their "illness" to a predecessor and to a family myth which they feel they have been compelled, in some helpless way, to follow.

Many theories of family life have been elaborated in recent years, most of them well beyond the range of this volume. Systems theorists, especially those in the field of family therapy, have described the inner workings of the family, focusing on interaction and communication. They have developed vocabularies to describe family patterns, the emotional and physical spaces families occupy, and the laws governing access to the dimensions of affect, power, and meaning in the family (Kantor and Lehr, 1975). Several workers have tried to develop a family typology (Fleck, 1980; Minuchin et al., 1967; Olson et al., 1979). Minuchin and his colleagues (1978) have advanced the concept of the "psychosomatic family." Bowen (1978) has put forth a model which emphasizes the three-generational development of symptoms or illness. Much of this innovative work has been well summarized by Hoffman (1981) and Walsh (1982).

The Mental Research Institute (MRI) group in Palo Alto, studying communications patterns in the families of schizophrenics, first developed concepts that meaningfully "fitted" identified patients' symptoms into their family dynamics (Bateson et al., 1956). Their work sparked interest in the patient's "illness" as a family phenomenon, and led to the work of others, especially Minuchin, who tried to characterize the family interactions of families with a psychosomatically ill member. Work with young diabetics and children with asthma or anorexia stimulated the further growth of interest in the interrelationship between illness and family factors.

At the same time, a number of physicians have observed links between family stress, such as the loss of a parent or a mate, and the onset or exacerbation of an illness (Grolnick, 1972; Huygen, 1982; Kellner, 1963; Klein et al., 1968; Kraus and Lilienfield, 1959; Parkes, 1972; Peachey, 1963). Earlier notions of psychosomatic illness have progressed well beyond their beginnings (Alexander, 1932; Dunbar, 1954) to consider the specific role of family stress in the appearance of illness symptomatology, as well as to examine the particular mechanisms by which stress is mediated, affecting especially the endocrine (Selye, 1956) and endocrinological (Locke, 1982) systems. As newer techniques become available today for studying the intricate workings of the immunological system, the physical mechanisms of stress become more available to study, thus finally offering a "bridge" to those seeking to understand how the body and mind work together to produce feelings, behavior, disease states, and so on.

In addition, researchers have begun to study the ways illness as an established fact impacts upon the family and forces it to alter its usual patterns.

The development of family medicine as a new specialty has further sharpened appreciation of the role of the family context around illness. This field surged into existence in the late 1960s, and is today the fastest-growing branch of U.S. medicine. Within the field, the notion of the family as the basic "unit of medical care" (Schmidt, 1978) has attracted a wide following, especially from physicians committed to a psychosocial orientation. Abetted by psychologists and social scientists who have been recruited into family medicine training programs, and whose orientation is opposed to the narrowly biomedical, family medicine has been able to explore how family factors both create and mitigate stress. A literature is thus emerging which looks at how the family and the illness affect one another (cf. the section on the relationship between illness and the family). Entire conferences and monographs have been devoted to the topic, and the development of the new journal *Family Systems Medicine* attests to the strength of the newly emerging paradigm.

Fundamental to this view is the conviction that one cannot grasp a patient's illness without understanding the social and emotional contexts in which he or she lives. This means inquiring into the family, work, school, community, ethnic, religious, etc., components of people's lives, because when people become sick their entire social network is often involved. One can see this, for example, in how people's social networks tend to condense around them to offer solace and support and to help them cope.

A systems approach leads one to understand the importance of many other subsystems when it comes to people's health—the role of workplace health hazards; the role of public health parameters such as sewage and water systems; the role of air pollution; the influence of prevailing cultural or community groups upon health practices such as fluoridation, contraception, alcoholism, and so on—yet no system other than the family carries an emotional burden or takes on continued responsibility for its members' well-being. The family engenders profound, lasting ties. In spite of its flaws and its problems, it has to be the central focus of a contextual approach (Worby, 1980) to illness behavior. More than any other system in which we live, the family serves as the context which defines, conditions, promotes, incites, affirms, negates, questions, softens, cares for, and otherwise creates the meaning of illness in our lives.

The physician encounters the patient's family in a number of ways. Family members have an unlimited capacity for suddenly materializing around a crisis, travelling hundreds of miles to be at the bedside of an ailing relative, phoning the physician for a word of advice or to offer their own explanation of what the problem "really" is. Similarly, the family can suddenly evaporate, split up and reassemble, create subgroups, hide one of its members from society, expel someone, and so on. Often, too, the family contains a "hidden patient," one whose problems are not brought to the physician, but whose disability or malfunction has affected the "identified patient." Often, too, as is well-known in family therapy circles, the "identified patient" is only a "signal," expressing the discord in the family and manifesting symptoms in response to family conflict. For example, an eight-year-old boy may be brought to the physician by his mother, with the complaint that he has "horrible pains in his stomach." Full "organic" workup may reveal "no pathology," and the problem may finally be appreciated as a "psychosomatic" or "functional" pain resulting from the sharp disputes between mother and father, which are creating tension in the son. In this case, to see the child as the "patient" and his pains as an "illness" only serves to mask what is really going on.

Further analysis of family behavior and family dynamics, especially as they affect illness, is beyond the scope of this section. Suffice it to say that the family, like any other open, living system, is capable of constant change, recurring pattern, equilibrium and disequilibrium, growth and decay. The patient is as embedded in the family as a tree in the earth, and cannot be fully understood apart from it.

THE MEDICAL SYSTEM

The physician belongs to the medical system, an enormous subunit of society involving millions and millions of people—physicians, nurses, hospital workers, clerks, paramedics, lab technicians, receptionists, X-ray personnel, and so on. This system is responsible for spending more than 12% of the U.S. gross national product. It extends towards other industries, too, such as the hospital supply corporations, drug companies, electronics concerns, and others.

Patients and their families come into contact with a great variety of these health workers in the course of their illness, any number of whom may deeply affect their lives. In the physician's office, for example, the patient or family member may become involved with the nurse, the receptionist, or the billing clerk. In the hospital, they may become involved with the nurse or orderly, the dietician, the medical student, the desk clerk, the supervisor, the administrator, and so on.

Any and all of these people intersect with the lives of patients and their families, and they may unexpectedly and profoundly influence the course of illness and its treatment. For example, one patient's wife was told by an orderly that her husband had less than a few weeks to live, whereas the physician had said nothing like that at all. Or again, the person who sweeps the floor may stop and comment to a patient, "What? You got myeloma? Jeez, my mother had that. It's a horrible disease. . . ."

A technician's offhand comment may agitate a patient for weeks; or, on the other hand, it may lead to a degree of solace not previously experienced. One woman was receiving an ultrasound exam to determine if her pregnancy was viable. The technician's comments that "it looks like the fetus is dead" kept the woman and her husband in a state of near-hysteria for two weeks. The physician was ignorant about the comment.

The medical system has its own rules, its own standards, and its own codes of behavior. Coming into contact with this monster at a time of perceived helplessness is sure to change and affect the patient's idea of the illness being experienced. The medical system is also a constant restraint and influence on the physician's behavior, for physicians must always be aware of others with somewhat conflicting interests (other generalists, specialists, utilization review committees, and the like) who look "over their shoulders."

Despite their vaunted independence, physicians are imbricated, one against the other, and jammed into a seething matrix of professional ties, rules, mores, relationships, and strains, all of which seek to determine their activity (cf. Freidson, 1970; Mechanic, 1978). What is the "usual standard of medical practice" but reflections of the physician's immersion in a system larger than himself?

The medical system itself interfaces with numerous other social systems—welfare, insurance companies, social security, disability, schools, courts, etc.—in ways which draw both patient and physician into contact with ever-widening systemic circles. For the purposes of this book, however, we will try to remain focused on the medical-family system interface, while understanding that each of these social units extends intimately towards other systems (workplace, schools, neighborhood, cultural group), and is not totally apart from any of them.

The patient-practitioner relationship takes place in this context, then. Yet, often the decisive factor in the patient's health-care picture is someone or something other than the physician supposes at first glance. It may, as in the following example, be the supervisor of homemaker placement in the local community:

Example 1

Mrs. P, an 84-year-old Russian-born Jewish widow living alone, presented in the office, sighing and in a state of near-collapse.

"Oy, doctor, you got a sick woman on your hands. My heart pounds. My head aches. I got a burnin' in my stomach that tears me apart. And my legs, my knees, they're all swollen up, I can't even walk. My knees, my hips. . . . And my digestion, a sour taste that I got in my mouth, the burning, and the gas. Oy! I don't know what I should do. I guess I'm a goner."

Her complaints were nothing new. But the degree of her incapacity was far beyond her usual state. For close to five minutes, she disgorged one complaint after another. She had burning in her stomach. Her chest ached. She couldn't see. She had no strength. She could barely walk. She lost her balance. Her knees were swollen. Her head throbbed. She was dizzy. Her back was stiff. She had gas. Her urine dribbled.

Finally, the conclusion of this odd recital emerged. ". . . And then they tell me I don't need my homemaker 15 hours a week.

They want to cut her back. And I just got out of the hospital three months ago. You should know whether I need her or not."

The occasion for her renewed complaints was the economy-minded supervisor's decision to trim her homemaker service; her subsequent rambling plea was for the physician, who had to be impressed by the alarming spread of all of her symptoms, to have the services reinstated.

The physician without a systemic perspective might have dismissed the woman as a "crock."

*   *   *

The foregoing example highlights a contextual approach to the patient-physician relationship. Often, the "chief complaint" is different from the medical "ticket" the patient has used to gain entry into the medical system. At other times, the family may be sending feelers to the medical system by bringing one of its members into it, in order to test the system's willingness to care.

A systemic approach attunes the physician to these other dimensions of the health-care encounter. Especially in the primary-care fields, the broader perspective deepens the grasp of why the patient has appeared, clarifies the likelihood of compliance, and hints at the significance of the encounter for the patient.

The traditional biomedical model has no place for such concerns, viewing them either as irrelevant or as hopelessly subjective and unscientific. Harassed and busy, the physician feels pleased to be able to grasp the "medical" problem at hand, let alone delve into its context. Yet, as has become increasingly clear, often the first is impossible without the second.

George Engel (1980) has provided a way for physicians to think about the different dimensions at which an illness operates (Figure 5). Using the example of a myocardial infarction, he shows how the patient's illness operates at the cellular level, the level of the organ and organ-system, and the level of the person, and how it affects the physicians, the hospital staff, the patient's spouse, the boss, and so on.

He comments:

> This stands in contrast to the orientation of the reductionist scientist, for whom confidence in the ultimate explanatory power of the factor-analytic approach in effect inhibits attention to what characterizes the whole. For medicine in particular the neglect of the whole . . . is largely responsible for the physician's preoccu-

pation with the body and with disease and the corresponding neglect of the patient as a person. (p. 538)

Such an approach blends the contemporary concern with the "whole
person" with older humanistic traditions of the family doctor. It reflects
the impact of social science upon medical practice and medical thought,
and thus brings practice towards a more interdisciplinary understanding. It is within this complex context that we approach the problem of
diagnosis today.

THE RELATIONSHIP BETWEEN ILLNESS AND THE FAMILY

People live in families, become ill in families, and are treated in their
family setting. As noted earlier, the influence of family factors on the
development and course of illness has recently become a topic of widespread and increasing interest. Much has been learned about this topic

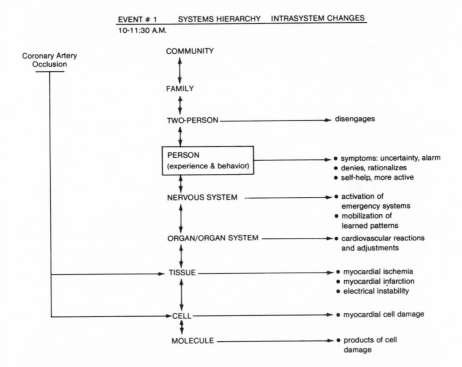

Figure 5. Systems analysis of a coronary artery occlusion (after Engel, 1980).

since the early review articles on the subject (Grolnick, 1972; Meissner, 1966).

In a way, it is amazing that medicine had gone on for years *without* going more deeply into the patient's family context. As Watzlawick et al. (1967) comment: "In modern biology, it would be unthinkable to study even the most primitive organism in artificial isolation from its environment" (p. 258). And yet this is what the biomedical model of illness has been doing for years.

Exceptions existed, of course. The early psychoanalysts were interested in childhood problems and often provided rich accounts of their patients' family life. General practitioners, who dealt with families for decades and who thus could observe evolving patterns of illness in ensuing generations, also commented on how families dealt with illness and on the relationship of illness to family stress (Kellner, 1963; Richardson, 1948); but their findings did not arouse much interest. Medicine was more intent on its growing specialization and tended to discount observations from astute family physicians, pediatricians, and other generalists.

The resurgence of family practice and the concurrent increased interest in illness among family therapists have given new impetus to the desire to understand illness in its family setting. Further scientific advances, especially from those working in the most biomedical of fields (such as immunology) have begun to clarify the role of stress in disease. To those who recognize the central role of the family as both a generator and a mediator of stress, the new biomedical findings cry out to be placed in some broader framework which can utilize them to relate stress, adaptation, and illness to people's psychosocial worlds.

Schmidt (1978), explaining the importance of taking the family as a basic unit of health care, notes that

> when providing primary medical care, there seems to be a definite advantage in centering this care about the family unit rather than the isolated individual patient. In other words, knowing what is 'going on' in the family seems to be equally as important as detailing the individual's symptoms. (p. 303)

He then lists several areas in which this approach seems productive:

1) the family's contribution to the "cause" of disease;
2) the family's contribution to the "cure" of disease;
3) the family's response to serious or chronic disease; and
4) the family's desire and/or need for family-oriented care.

Such a perspective rests on several assumptions. First, it assumes that emotional stress affects illness (the "psychosomatic premise"). Second, it assumes that symptoms, in fact all illness behavior, are understandable: Their meaning emerges and becomes clearer when seen in the context in which they develop. Finally, it assumes that, as an illness develops, it affects the patient and his or her family, and is affected by them in turn: the "two-way" hypothesis. Many studies have shown that these assumptions are correct. Their sum result is to expand the physician's frame of reference from a one-person field to the family (and broader social) field.

ORIGINS OF A FAMILY SOMATIC APPROACH

The roots of this perspective can be traced to three sources:

1) Psychoanalysis, a fervid, creative intellectual force for decades, which understood that behavior had roots in family process and whose theoreticians began to explore the family contexts of illness. It was psychoanalysis which in fact spawned the fields of psychosomatic medicine and family therapy.
2) The development of modern stress theory by Cannon (1920) and Selye (1956), which provided scientific basis for exploring the mechanisms involved in stress-related illness.
3) The decades of work in psychosomatic medicine, which kept insisting that the mind/body split was in our own minds, not in the workings of nature, and that all illnesses had to be perceived in a more holistic way than medicine was doing at that time.

The movement was further abetted by other factors. These included:

1) the tradition of social medicine as another discipline committed to seeing illness in its broader, social context—this had gained strength from developments in social psychology, medical sociology, and related social sciences; and
2) the tradition of family (general) practice (cf. Huygen, 1982), which consistently provided a concrete world of experience and data for analysis and reflection.

Decades ago, Kanner (1948) examined the transmission of parental hypochondriasis to their children, and Goldberg (1958) and Garner and Weinar (1959) both examined family influences in the so-called psychosomatic disorders. Bruch, exploring obesity and other eating disorders (1973), moved from a strictly psychoanalytical to include a family-oriented perspective.

The trend received a tremendous boost from the growth of family therapy in the past 20 years. The group at Palo Alto's Mental Research Institute, including Gregory Bateson, Jay Haley, Don Jackson, Paul Watzlawick, and John Weakland, developed an understanding of family communication patterns which they initially applied to the symptoms of the (identified) schizophrenic. They extended this understanding to other forms of behavior, and soon Weakland (1977) prophetically declared that all symptoms, even physical illness, might productively be regarded simply as behavior.

These insights led to working with the family context of a large number of physical illnesses. Therapists moved from investigating schizophrenic children to working with diabetic youngsters, asthmatics, and anorectics. Soon almost all the traditional psychosomatic disorders were being pursued from a family perspective, which included interactional, psychodynamic, and communicational features.

Principal among these workers was Salvador Minuchin and his group in Philadelphia. Coining the term "psychosomatic families" (1978), these authors showed how attention to family dynamic patterns could clarify the course of many psychosomatic illnesses.

This line of investigation dovetailed into observations from mainstream general practice and pediatrics, many of which of course dealt with the observed effects of family stress on the appearance and subsequent course and management of illness.

In 1948 the monograph *Patients Have Families* appeared. Authored by Henry B. Richardson, a general practitioner, this work was the report of a two-year interdisciplinary study funded by the Josiah Macy, Jr. Foundation in New York City. The group studied 15 families, with the goal of understanding "the interrelation between illness and the family situation." This book included the notion of the family as a "system" and as a "unit of illness," and concluded by asking practitioners to consider "the family in all its complexities." One chapter of the book dealt with the cooperation between psychiatrist and (medical) physician in dealing with the different aspects of illness in a family setting. Such an approach now appears to have been 30 years ahead of its time.

Fifteen years later, in England, the general practitioner Robert Kellner published *Family Ill Health* (1963). This was a report on 346 families in a British general practice. Kellner found that

1) chronic and recurrent illness in one family member had a strong effect on the health of the others;
2) an outbreak of physical illness in one family member was commonly followed by the aggravation of a mild neurosis in another; and
3) a wife's illness followed a husband's more than twice as often as the reverse.

Kellner realized that illness in the family could lead to unhappiness, neurotic symptoms, psychosomatic illness, and even physical illness in other family members. He conjectured, too, that some visits to the doctor were occasioned by reasons other than the announced complaint, and he urged physicians to be more aware of such phenomena.

Other physicians were attracted by patterns in the way some families utilized the resources of their physician. Peachey (1963), focusing on a three-year period of general practice with 25 families, showed four types of attendance patterns: 1) constant illness, 2) regular periodicity, 3) clustering, and 4) simultaneity. She hypothesized that families have definite patterns of illness, and that such patterning is characteristic of a particular family. Furthermore, insofar as they suggest possible contributing etiologic agents and serve to predict further dysfunction, the patterns may offer guides for both treatment and prevention.

Many investigators have looked at the effects of the loss of loved ones, especially a wife or husband. Over and over, the loss of a spouse has been shown to be linked with a greater susceptibility to illness of all types, and to death. This is especially true for men.

Kraus and Lilienfield's classic study (1959) explored the markedly elevated mortality rate among 30-35-year-old, recently widowed men. They observed that "the excess risk in the widowed under 35, compared to the married, was greater than tenfold for at least one of the specific age-sex groups, involving several leading causes of death" (p. 217).

This observation was followed in the next decade by a number of important papers. Kreitman (1964) and Klein et al. (1968) showed that the devastation visited on the surviving spouse by the death of the loved one included the appearance of physical illness. Young et al. (1963) and Rees and Lutkins (1967) both investigated the "mortality of bereavement." The former found that death rates increased over 40% during the first six months of bereavement. The latter, examining over 900 close relatives of 371 residents of a Welsh community who died over a five-year period, found that almost 5% died within a year of being bereaved, compared to 0.7% for a control group.

The topic of bereavement has formed the focus of over two decades of work by Colin Parkes, whose work (1972) is the classic in the field. Similar findings, accompanied by a reflective look at the meaning and medical consequences of loneliness, appear in *The Broken Heart* by James J. Lynch (1979).

Research has gone into infectious disease as well. Meyer and Haggerty (1962), pursuing susceptibility to streptococcal infections, found that 37% were associated with a form of acute stress. In addition, incidence rose in families with "high" chronic family stress, as compared to those with "low" chronic stress. Dingle and his co-workers (1964) showed that the incidence of simple respiratory illness varies according to family relationship. Recently, Patterson (1983) has addressed the notion of chronic *strain*, rather than "stress" in general, as a stressor of family life.

In a now classic study, Medalie et al. (1973) found that, among men subject to arteriosclerotic cardiovascular disease, "psychosocial factors" were as significant a risk factor for developing angina pectoris as was hypertension or the blood cholesterol level. The weight of psychosocial factors was greater than that of cigarette smoking in predicting the development of angina. Others have confirmed this finding; subsequently, discussion has been intense about the role of the "Type A personality" (Friedman, 1969) in the development of cardiovascular disease, especially angina and myocardial infarction.

Psychosomatic medicine has examined the relationship between stress and illness, although it has not yet focused sharply on the family as the main source of stress and the main context for evolving illness (cf. Lipowski et al., 1977, for an excellent, up-to-date textbook in this field). Researchers now are beginning to explain the different types of stress families in trouble experience, thus laying the foundation for the approach to the new terrain John Weakland dubbed "family somatics" (1977).

In addition, psychoimmunologists have begun explaining how stress affects the immune system. This has implications not only for diseases such as allergy, cancer, many types of infections—ranging from herpes, mononucleosis, and strep throat—and the auto-immune illness, but also for almost any other sickness as well. The recent appearance of the textbook *Psychoneuroimmunology* (Ader, 1982) goes a long way to develop this entire field. Once the biochemical, physiological reactions can be understood, it is but a matter of time before investigators can observe families in their normal routine and assess how "normal" stress predisposes to or promotes illness. (For a discussion of what is normal, see Froma Walsh's introductory chapter in Walsh, 1982.)

This topic, growing so rapidly it can only be touched upon briefly here, provides for study of the "missing link" in the psychosomatic explanation—the actual physical workings of stress. Such developments carry profound significance for the notion of diagnosis.

Recent work by Huygen (1982) has provided a rich amount of data and insight. Physicians must now be aware of several types of situations in which knowledge of the family is imperative:

- A first is when the family appears to be harboring, generating, or promoting the illness of one of its members.
- A second is when an illness intrudes so suddenly, so cataclysmally, upon a family that it needs help in orienting itself to the stress and coping with it.
- A third is when chronic illness appears to be relapsing uncontrollably.
- A fourth is when compliance seems to be an issue defying the physician's control.
- A fifth is when an illness appears to be psychosomatic or stress-related, but the index patient admits of no problem or concern.
- A sixth is when the family members phone the physician repeatedly to offer secret information which they insist cannot be relayed on to the patient.
- A seventh is when a child or other member of the family appears to be getting ill in the context of severe conflict between two other members.
- An eighth is when death touches a family.

Illness affects family dynamics and is affected by them. Families, for example, usually have rules determining how intense pain must be before anyone will grant it legitimacy, how intense it must be before anyone will be brought to a physician. Rules promote or interdict different diagnoses, and they control access to the medical system.

Family rules also define what a "good" physician's response to an illness is, and what constitutes adequate care. Families usually have a sense of which member(s) is the patient in the family, and which member(s) are caretakers, secret sufferers, or will be hidden from the medical system entirely.

Families also share myths of different illnesses. They pass images of

On Diagnosis

illness down from generation to generation. These meaningful constructs influence patienthood, the creation and appearance of illness, family response to sickness, compliance with medical regimes, and the actual felt experience of any particular illness.

In sum, the interrelationship between illness and the family is a two-way street, extending through all phases of an illness and through all stages of family life. Practitioners will find that a contextual perspective helps clarify their work with almost any patient, and with virtually any difficult problem.

CHAPTER 5

The Phenomenology of Diagnosis

BEFORE THE SYSTEMS MEET

Diagnoses can be established in a number of ways. Many forms of diagnoses, for example, never reach the medical system. As Freidson has pointed out (1970), patients are ensconced in a rich world of their own, marked by its own ethnic, class, and cultural values. Medical advice often comes from friends and relatives. In addition, many cultural and ethnic groups have lay healers who treat a number of quasi-medical problems which never come to a physician's attention.

Many people who experience pain, for example, will speak to a friend or relative about it first, before heading to a doctor. Often, in fact, a referral to a doctor takes place only after the patient's complaints and worry are validated by someone else, who approves of the referral. Many times, the friend will direct the patient to a particular doctor, folk healer, druggist, and so on.

The initial step in diagnosis, before it draws the attention of the medical system, can be called *self-diagnosis*. Patients feel ill, out of sorts, and unlike themselves. "Something is wrong," they decide. Usually, they will try to figure out if it is "something" or "nothing." The former will need attention; the latter will probably go away by itself. People faced with a set of disagreeable and aggravating bodily complaints may conclude, "I think it's my stomach acting up again. I hope it's not an ulcer.

43

I'd better watch what I eat for a few days and see." Or they may say, "Hmm. This seems like a case of nerves. I'd better try to relax. Maybe I should take some Maalox." Or again, "Oh no, I hope this isn't an ulcer like my dad had!"

Many self-diagnosed complaints, having reached this level, go no further. The patient (let us call the afflicted person that, for want of a better uniformly identifying term) takes a home remedy or some other form of treatment. He or she gets better, or decides to accept and/or ignore the problem unless it gets worse.

Much of people's lives is spent worrying about the little aches and pains which seem unusual, perhaps the mark of some disease. Tolstoy's Ivan Illich and Sartre's Roquentin suffer existential anxiety over somatic symptoms, which they keep to themselves. The significance of the symptom is usually hidden, even from the sufferers themselves, who worry all alone, building explanations in their own mind why this or that symptom should be afflicting them.

When the person who feels ill asks a friend or relative for advice, it often leads to what can be termed *peer-diagnosis*. Interactions with the local pharmacist, an uncle, a cousin who happens to be a nurse, a minister, a salesman, the kid next door—each of these may produce a conviction that the symptoms are indeed important, and that the person is suffering from some kind of illness. The friend may, on the other hand, help to dismiss the symptom with a phrase or two: "Take it easy." "Don't worry." "Take an afternoon off."

Depending on the involved lay culture, its values and its array of available lay healers, the potential patient is usually pointed in one or another direction: towards a herbal cure, a fad food diet, an osteopath, a faith healer, a whole health center, a natural foods store, or even (as sometime occurs) a physician.

He may be told: "Gee, I don't know what you've got, Chuck, but it sounds exactly like what my brother Sam had last year. Why don't you go see Dr. Caravalho? He helped Sam out a lot." Or: "Brenda, it just sounds like a case of nerves. Maybe you're eating too much sugar." Or: "My sister's a nurse, and she says *everyone* is taking Vitamin E for that. . . ."

In spite of the ubiquity of self-diagnosis and peer-diagnosis, however, diagnosis as a legitimate phenomenon does not occur until the patient contacts the physician or some other representative of the medical system. The remainder of this discussion will focus on encounters of this type, in which people who wonder if they are ill come to the attention of physicians capable of officially diagnosing the problem and giving them an answer.

BALINT'S CONTRIBUTION

Michael Balint, a British psychoanalyst who worked for years with groups of general practitioners, described how diagnoses were established in his classic *The Doctor, His Patient, and the Illness* (1957). This monograph, which has been said to have "changed the face of British medicine" (Obituary, 1971), applies a contextual and humanistic perspective to the doctor-patient encounter, and is grounded in a sensitive appreciation of that interaction. It is must reading for every student of the topic.

The entire first part of Balint's work addresses the question of diagnosis. So germinal is its analysis that any subsequent discussion must begin with what Balint says.

He begins by analyzing what happens when the doctor and the patient meet. The two parties start to "negotiate" the diagnosis:

> The patient in his still "unorganized" state [makes] various "offers" of illness to his doctor, and the doctor [responds] to these offers by rejecting some of them and finally accepting one. An important aspect of the doctor's response is the process of "elimination by appropriate physical examinations" resulting in the establishment of a ranking order both of illnesses and of patients. Under the impact of the doctor's response, a kind of "agreement" is more often than not reached between him and the patient, and the illness thus enters upon its "organized" phase. (p. 107)

Feeling poorly and wondering why this is so, the patient approaches the physician for advice. Patients may have their own ideas of what is wrong. They may present certain symptoms rather than others in an effort to feel out the physician's responsiveness to their distress. They often have their own agendas which determine how they will maneuver. But in any case, they will present a set of complaints which form "offers" in Balint's terminology: invitations to a working diagnosis. The physician may accept or reject these offers. At this stage the illness is said to be "unorganized." It does not yet have a name. There is no diagnosis. The doctor and patient may proceed in any of a number of directions. There is much to be said for keeping this phase of the illness "open" as long as possible, especially if the physician senses that the presentation is complex.

The patient then offers another set of symptoms and/or complaints, requests, or suggestions. At some point, the physician "accepts" one of these offers, or he makes a counter-offer which the patient then accepts ("No, I don't think this is indigestion at all. It may very well be your gall bladder."); the illness becomes named and thus enters upon its "organized" phase. The diagnosis is beginning to crystallize.

At this point, treatment may officially begin, although often it will have started earlier, and its results may even have helped contribute to the agreed-upon diagnosis.

Example 2

Philip C, a 32-year-old married accountant, came to the physician complaining of horrible burning in his stomach. He was afraid of an ulcer, "just like my father had." In good health all his life, he had recently been under increasing stress at work, and was starting to squabble with his wife at home. At the initial encounter, the history of his symptoms was taken, and a complete physical exam was performed. Because the patient was so worried about the possibility of an ulcer, an upper GI series was ordered, and the patient was given a prescription for a mild anti-spasmodic medication. "It could be an ulcer, of course," the physician said. "But it could just as well be a couple of other things, including the effects of stress on your stomach. We'll see."

The second session a week later found the patient feeling better. The X-ray study was normal, as were the routine blood tests. The physician and patient discussed both the work situation and the squabbles at home, and the physician explained some of the effects of stress on the stomach. The medication was continued.

By the third session, two weeks later, the patient's symptoms had dwindled markedly. "I'm able to figure out when the spasms will start," he said. The anti-spasmodic medication was continued for another three months, and was then tapered. Both patient and physician agreed on the diagnosis of a stress-related stomach condition.

Balint goes on to describe physicians' frequent bias against considering emotional factors (he calls them "neurotic symptoms") as main contributors to patients' distress. Instead, physicians are prone to emphasize physical illness instead, most likely because they feel more comfortable with it. Afraid of missing a "real illness," physicians often proceed by "eliminating" one medical possibility after another by virtue of physical exams, X-ray studies, tests, probes, biopsies, CT scans, and so on. One consequence of this bias, of course, is that the patient becomes fixed in viewing his or her problem as mainly physical, and thus resists efforts to understand it in context.

Physicians still go through a similar process today. In fact, the most sophisticated physicians draw up a list of "differential" diagnostic possibilities, which incorporate the different possible diseases the patient's symptoms might represent. Instead of proceeding from the most likely to the lesser possibilities, physicians in training are often rewarded for thinking of the most abstruse possibilities, and for ordering the (expensive!) tests which rule out such options. Students are trained to "think of zebras when you hear hoofbeats" by such erudite exercises as the instructive Clinical Pathological Conference printed weekly in the *New England Journal of Medicine*, where the correct anatomical-pathological diagnosis is often quite rare.

Balint disagrees with the usual approach. He feels "there is a danger, not only in missing a physical sign, but also in finding one" (p. 62), especially if it diverts attention from more important factors which affect the patient's symptoms. His point is simple, but direct: If the likelihood of emotional disorder is very high, don't waste a lot of time pursuing lesser possibilities, if you can possibly help it. The patient will be the one to suffer if you do.

His view, in fact, has much in common with some recent work discussing medical decisions. The work follows a triage pattern, and is affected by the "probabilistic model" (Bursztjan et al., 1981). The point is first to eliminate those diseases which are potentially life-threatening, especially if they are treatable. Then one proceeds to the most likely diagnostic possibility and uses it as a working hypothesis. Such patterns of decision-making have, in fact, been proposed, but have not caught on in the academic centers.

The more important emotional issues form the substance of what Balint refers to as the "deeper level of diagnosis." This relates the patient's symptoms (and even the patient's illness) to the patient's context—family life, past memories, fears, worries, personality patterns, and so on. In this sense Balint's concern with this "deeper level" forms a well-reasoned brief for the physician's dealing with the "whole person" rather than with a set of symptoms. Balint's (1957) arguments seem ahead of their time:

> We must realize that in general practice the real problem is often the illness of the whole person—as every medical student has had preached to him on innumerable occasions . . . (p. 39). It is advisable for the doctor to aim at a more comprehensive, deeper diagnosis. By this I mean a diagnosis which is not content with comprehending all the physical signs and symptoms, but [which] tries to evaluate the pertinence of the so-called "neurotic" symptoms. (p. 55)

The deeper level of diagnosis addresses itself to the patient's family and social situation, as well as to his or her past history and "psychodynamics." It foreshadows what Engel (1977) refers to as the biopsychosocial model, and what Worby (1980) has termed "contextual medicine."

Concern for this often-missed dimension of patients' distress led Balint to propose "long sessions" to physicians. These are one- or two-hour-long encounters with the patient (although certainly not, in current use, limited to the doctor and patient alone) in the course of which the physician tries to explore the context of the patient's complaints and better grasp their inner significance. One long session may prevent many fruitless visits for psychosomatic complaints that do not improve, or that move from organ system to organ system in familiar, frustrating patterns.

Example 3

Sally H, an attractive, 25-year-old divorcee, visited the doctor complaining of odd aches in her legs and thighs. She felt her veins were "popping out." Sometimes her legs felt hot and flushed, throbbing. A friend had told her she might have "phlebitis," and, as her mother had been ill for years with that condition, she was quite distraught.

Physical examination was totally negative. Her veins did not bulge at all. If anything, the physician noted her to be quite anxious and somewhat seductive.

On the second visit, the patient continued to insist, in a most obsessing manner, that she might have phlebitis. So agitated was she, in fact, that a venogram was finally ordered, along with a vascular surgery consultation. The venogram report was delayed: The patient insisted the technician had said it was "positive" and phoned twice in an exceedingly agitated state. Yet the report came back—normal. The vascular surgeon said he found "no pathology," agreed that she seemed quite anxious, and suggested . . . an orthopedic referral!

By the third visit, the patient complained of feeling worried because "nobody can find out what's wrong." She announced a decision to visit a chiropractor. She denied being upset at anything else in her life, but on further discussion it was obvious that she was overwhelmed trying to cope with a number of job-related, financial, and personal issues all at once. She was divorced and having trouble with her son. Her parents did not approve of how she was living. And so on.

A "long session" was offered her in hopes of getting a better sense of the context in which her rather vague and confusing symptoms had emerged. The hour was spent discussing her family life, from her early years through the dissolution of her marriage and her struggle to get on her feet financially. At the end of the session, she again raised her symptoms and was prescribed a simple anti-inflammatory medication and advised to return in a week. She accepted the formulation that perhaps the swelling and pain in her legs were due to a minor muscle pull, which was being aggravated by stress.

At the next visit, she said her pains were somewhat less, but she was now having warm flushed feelings in her legs. The physician asked her about feelings of sexual excitation, and commented that congestion of the blood vessels in the pelvic area, as occurs when sexual feelings are not discharged, is sometimes associated with such throbbing sensations. She accepted the comment with some surprise, and later agreed that, whatever the cause of her symptoms, it did not seem to be a serious problem, would probably get better, and that stress and worry were making it worse. The illness was yet far from being "organized," but the long session had laid the groundwork for a more open and all-sided relationship.

Balint spent a good deal of time, too, discussing the physician's response to the patient, and explaining how it can provide clues to the final diagnosis. Such insights are gained from applying the notions of transference and countertransference to the medical encounter, and exploring how the physician's feelings and responses shed light on the patient's own personality patterns. This topic moves away from us here, but is a fascinating aspect of the clinician's use of self as a diagnostic tool.

In sum, then, Balint gives us a description of the doctor-patient encounter as it develops into a relationship, and speaks of the different aspects of the diagnostic process. In family practice, where close to 75% of the care is concerned, at least in part, with the emotional aspects of the patient and the family's life, Balint's writings keep us alert to the different dimensions of patients' distress, and point us always in the "deeper" direction of ascertaining the symptoms' significance and meaning for that particular patient.

THE TIP OF THE ICEBERG: THE DOCTOR-PATIENT RELATIONSHIP

The doctor-patient relationship is universally acknowledged as the cornerstone of medical care. Our orientation here is to view this encounter as a special example of the interaction between the medical and family (or social) systems. To be sure, the intensity and life-and-death concerns of the doctor-patient relationship make it unique, in ways which can be elsewhere addressed in their own right. For our purposes here, however, in understanding how a diagnosis is made and what it means, we will try to adhere to a more comprehensive, systemic perspective.

Parsons' View

The systemic understanding of this relationship has its 20th-century beginnings with Lawrence Henderson's article, "Physician and patient as a social system" (1935). Henderson, remembered by many for his role in developing the Henderson-Hasselbach equation, was originally a biochemist who turned towards sociology. He taught a course in "Concrete Sociology" at Harvard, where one of his students was Talcott Parsons.

While Henderson focused on the internal workings of the doctor-patient relationship, Parsons delved into the social roles of both patient and practitioner. Parsons' writings form the basis for today's analysis of the doctor-patient relationship. He saw the relationship as a necessary feature of society, patterned and regulated so it can be useful. According to Parsons, the relationship rests on a basic mutuality of needs and outlook. Physicians are especially trained in their area of expertise. Patients come to them seeking help. The relationship is inherently unequal. Patients are dependent, all the more so because illness often brings about a state of helplessness and regression. They are thus compelled to take on "the sick role," which places them in a well-defined social position.

According to Parsons, this role has four characteristics:

1) Patients cannot be held responsible for their incapacity.
2) Their illness is a legitimate excuse from their usual social obligations.
3) In order to merit these excuses, patients must want to get well.
4) Towards this end, they must seek competent medical advice and cooperate with their physicians.

Freidson, reviewing this (1970), has commented—a bit more wryly than Parsons—that "medicine creates the social possibilities for acting sick."

The practitioner's role in the Parsonian model is a functionally specialized, full-time activity, attained through special training which has imparted a minimum standard of professional competence. Practitioners must also adopt an attitude of "affective neutrality" towards their patients. This means approaching patients objectively, and not letting subjective feelings interfere with professional judgment. Affective neutrality is physicians' main safeguard against using patients for their own interests—sexually, financially, politically, and so on. It is the patients' guarantee, too, and thus forms a cornerstone of the professional relationship.

Two other cardinal dimensions of the professional attitude, according to Parsons, are its "universality" and "functional specificity." The former means that physicians treat *all* their patients in the same way, without bias or judgment; the second means that they limit their professional activity to what they have been trained to do.

All this implies a fundamental unity of interest between patient and practitioner, whose relationship is thus neat, mutual, and complementary.

Critiques of the Parsonian View

Many sociologists have challenged Parsons' view. Eliot Freidson, for example, influenced by the "social constructivist" school of sociology, exposes the potential for conflict latent in the encounter. Rather than focusing on the supposed mutuality of the patient-practitioner relationship, Freidson delves into its hostility, ambivalence, and clash of cultural and class perspective.

According to him, medicine is "engaged in the construction of illness as a social state which a human being may assume" (1970, p. 205). Medicine's monopoly includes "the right to create illness as an official social role" (p. 206). The patient's sense of being ill is not legitimized until the physician makes his or her diagnosis. In this lies the seeds of conflict—for patients and physicians each come from different worlds, and each brings different values, needs, hierarchies, and agendas:

> Diagnosis and treatment are not biological acts common to mice, monkeys, and men, but [are] social acts peculiar to men. Illness as such may be biological disease, but the idea of illness is not, and neither is the way human beings respond to it. Thus biological deviance or disease is defined socially and is surrounded by social acts that condition it. (Freidson, 1970, p. 209)

This understanding leads Freidson to explore the *context* of illness, the meanings attributed to physical illness by patient and physician, and the motivations physicians often attribute to patients' behavior. He also criticizes Parsons' neglect of chronic or permanent illness.

In examining the "professional construction of illness," Freidson brings out physicians' own class interest and self-interest. Mainly in private practice, most physicians can be regarded as "moral entrepreneurs," trafficking in illness as a social commodity. This leads them at times to overdiagnose or overtreat.

Freidson also points out that there are different kinds of doctor-patient relationships. For our purposes, this has a strong impact on the kinds of diagnoses reached. One type of relationship, typical of primary care and family practice, is called "client-dependent." In this kind of practice, the patient is self-referred to the physician, or perhaps referred by someone else in his own family or social group. The other kind of patient-practitioner relationship is typified by the interaction between patients and specialists, what Freidson calls "colleague-dependent." Here, the patient comes to the physician usually through the referral activity of some other physician. (In this sense, many generalists are called "feeders" by specialists, who rely on them for their income.)

Because the primary-care physician tends to see the patient over a longer time, and thus to know the patient in his or her family setting, the patient in this kind of relationship actually has more clout, more impact, in that the physician is more likely to listen to him or her, is more *responsive* to his or her wishes.

Specialist-consultants, on the other hand, have little to gain from catering to the patient's wishes. Their main duty is to give the referring physician a correct appraisal of the patient's problems. The better the consultant note, the more likely is the referring physician to continue to refer.

One feature of changing medical practice today is the number of self-referred patients who approach the medical specialist. In a sense, doing this already presupposes that a diagnosis has been reached. And, certainly, going to a skin doctor with a rash, or to a pulmonary physician with trouble breathing, or to an orthopedist with hip pain, points the physician in the direction of diagnosing "within his discipline." One function family physicians provide is to act as ombudsmen for their patients, taking the responsibility to refer them to the appropriate specialist. That is, someone with cardiac-based difficulty breathing will not be referred to a fellow in pulmonary medicine used to treating chronic lung disease.

A problem emerges when specialists emancipate themselves from dependence on the primary-care physician, a phenomenon which appears to be occurring in several ways. On the one hand, many physicians who work in large teaching diagnostic centers and hospitals practice specialty medicine, and do not need physician-referrals, since their patients are triaged by the house officers towards the appropriate specialty clinics. On the other hand, the development of some HMO's has led to a broad panel of specialist care, masquerading as primary-care medicine. (The Harvard Community Health Plan, for example, has no family practitioners, but it does have a selection of pediatricians, internists, ob-gynecologists, and so on.) Patients who join these HMO's may wind up with specialists who are practicing primary care. Similarly, many young specialists have now taken positions in the community, whereby they practice primary-care medicine in their offices but are also responsible for specialty medical clinics in the local hospital, for a fixed salary.

The strength of Freidson's analysis is his exploration of the practitioner's everyday world. Differences between doctors and patients, and between different doctors and different patients, are grounded in their different stations in life, their different self-interests. The medical encounter means different things to its participants. For example, as Elihu Gerson (1976) has noted, medicine is both the physician's way of making a living and a "grossly uncomfortable, often painful, often embarrassing, frequently terrorizing experience" (p. 219) for the patient. Such profound difference adds tension to the encounter.

Different values lead to different expectations for the encounter. Many physicians "medicalize" the doctor-patient time, using it to search for symptoms, signs of illness, and treatment issues. Patients, who are immersed in a world of social obligation, know the value of a well-written doctor's note when the chips are down. But here is where the conflict develops. Sometimes, for example, the patient wants a prescription or a note for work, but the physician does not want to give it. In this case, the supposed mutuality of the relationship crumbles as the two parties struggle for control.

Example 4

Peggy F, a 45-year-old divorced woman with one child, drops by the physician's office after having been absent from the practice for a year. She complains of pains in her back and "incidentally" wishes to "drop off" a form for welfare certification.

She is about 150 pounds overweight, and has been "unable" to lose any of it. She has claimed "terrific" arthritis pains in her spine, even though X-rays have shown "minimal" degenerative changes.

Her only previous job has been as a taxicab driver, but she claims she cannot work anymore in that capacity because of her persistent backache.

Leafing through the chart, the physician notes numerous missed appointments, failure to comply with prescribed medications, and requests for sedatives and sleeping pills. The physician feels angry, "conned." "There is really no evidence in the chart here," he begins, "to substantiate that your back has any *serious* damage. Why even the X-rays . . ."

"I'm in *agony*, doc," Peggy says, cutting in and moving her position as if preparing for a fight. "Don't you *believe* me?"

In any busy family practice, patients come to the physician for many reasons, some of which the physician may not particularly sympathize with. For example, when a patient wants a disability certificate, the physician—even when he has known the patient for some time—may feel that the patient is a "shirker," in spite of his avowed intent to treat the patient "objectively." And, having feelings about the use and abuse of public revenue in welfare and disability causes, he may make these views clear to the patient. Very clearly, the physician only does what he feels "honest" in doing; being untrue to his own moral, ethical and social prejudices feels "dishonest."

Parsons' (1951) pose of affective neutrality, then, is actually most possible when the patient and the physician share class and cultural background. The further apart they are, the greater the chance that their agendas will differ. The results of the ensuing disappointment are found in the growing accounts of patients' anger and disillusion with their physicians, their denunciations of physician affluence, and their crusade for more available, compassionate, and caring physicians.

Much of this criticism may actually confuse contemporary physicians. They feel they are trained, after all, to diagnose and treat their patients' illnesses, not to be their minister or friend. (The old-time GP is not a model for today's young medical student.) The physician's gripe is that patients tend to be "uppity" these days, asking too many questions, rushing for second opinions, suing for malpractice at the drop of a hat, and failing to follow the simplest and most reasonable forms of medical advice.

The Battle for Control

While Parsons presents the physician as benevolent and kindly, trying to help patients cope with their distress, Waitzkin and Stoeckle (1976) identify the physician as an instrument of social control. According to them, physicians transmit society's prevalent cultural and moral values, and are thus representatives of the dominant class in any given society.

Others (Mishler et al, 1981; Szasz, 1974; Illich, 1976) have described the physician's role in isolating groups of social "deviants" from the rest of society. This process has concerned the contagiously ill (Foucault, 1965), the morally degenerate or hopelessly insane (Szasz, 1974), and so on. They have pointed out the problems which come up in using illness to label people. Consider the following as medical "illnesses": homosexuality, menopause, pregnancy, alcoholism, frigidity, impotence, contraceptive counseling, child abuse, adolescent stress reaction, senility, school phobia, etc. Much focuses around the question of control, and around the hierarchy established in the patient-practitioner relationship. How equal are the two parties? Which has the power to make the other act?

An excellent analysis around this issue comes from (once again) Szasz, who wrote an article with Hollander (1956) dealing with different models of the doctor-patient relationship. They describe three models (Figure 6):

a) The model of *activity-passivity* is at one extreme. The physician is active; the patient, passive. The best example of this is when the patient is in a coma and the doctor acts to save his life. The basic model of this relationship is the way a parent relates to a child.

b) The model of *guidance-cooperation* is very close to the Parsonian model. Here, the caring physician tells the patient what is best, and the

Model	Physician's role	Patient's role	Clinical application of model	Prototype of model
Activity-passivity	Does something to patient	Recipient (unable to respond or inert)	Anesthesia, acute trauma, delirium, coma, etc.	Parent-infant
Guidance-cooperation	Tells patient what to do	Cooperator (obeys)	Acute infectious processes, etc.	Parent-child (adolescent)
Mutual participation	Helps patient to help himself	Participant in "partnership" (uses expert help)	Most chronic illnesses, psychoanalysis, etc.	Adult-adult

Figure 6. The three basic models in the Szasz-Hollander conceptualization of the doctor-patient relationship.*

*From Szasz, T.S., and Hollander, M.H.: Arch. Intern. Med. **97**:585-592, 1956. Copyright 1956 by the American Medical Association.

patient follows advice. To some degree, the patient exercises some control, but basically the ("good") patient is the one who follows the doctor's orders.

c) The model of *mutual participation*, advocated by Szasz and Hollander, involves the patient much more actively. Here the patient is an eager participant, who uses the doctor's opinion as part of the basis for making up his or her own mind. The basic model of this relationship is of two adults, open and sharing.

While Szasz and Hollander appear to idealize the degree of mutuality capable of being found in this relationship—after all, the doctor *is* the expert, which is why the patient came to the office in the first place—the gamut of actual doctor-patient relationships certainly follows what they suggest. Physicians vary on a spectrum of activity and authoritarianism. So do patients. Some patients prefer being told what to do. (I am thinking here of many Italian patients who, on being asked which option they prefer to follow, often exclaim with dismay, "I don't know. If I knew, I wouldn't have come to you. You tell me what to do, and I'll do it. *You're* the doctor." Physicians concerned with respecting their patients' rights to their own opinions will also have to respect their right to want to be told what to do. Here, the physician who gives advice is actually following the patient's directive. The phenomenon is not at all simple.)

Some patients, of course, appreciate being given a chance to help make their own decisions. Other patients positively insist on it or have family members who insist on it, regardless of the doctor's advice. (This position, incidentally, is not recognized in the Szasz-Hollander formulation, a point which Hingson et al., 1981, also make.)

At any rate, it is clear that the pleasant mutuality of the Parsonian model breaks down repeatedly when faced with differences between physician and patient or between their expectations of the encounter. The questions of who is controlling the relationship and whose idea it is that that person is in control are not unimportant. Here is where the Parsonian model falters, and a model which understands conflict becomes more helpful.

Example 5

Mary T, a strong-willed woman in her forties, announces to the physician on her very first visit that her previous physician did not respect her, that he told her what to do and did not listen to her, and that she has left him for that reason. Her medical problems include hypertension and pelvic pains and infections. She says she has her own ideas about the treatment she needs. She expects to make all her own decisions.

The physician feels instantly put upon and manipulated, uneasy. He feels that the other physician is being torn down as someone who didn't care and who didn't listen, and envisages that—in another three months—the patient will be telling this same story to yet another physician. He hears Mary say she wants to make her own decisions, *so he decides to let her make her own decisions* in order to keep her as a patient for the time being. So long as a decision is not deleterious, in his view, he will not oppose it.

The two of them have now, at the patient's instigation, mutually agreed to let the patient make her main treatment decisions. There is nothing unusual or paradoxical about this. It happens every day.

BENEATH THE TIP OF THE ICEBERG: SYSTEMS IN INTERACTION

The preceding discussion leads to viewing a patient's illness in a broader context. Once this takes place, physicians usually find that the existing diagnostic labels are inadequate. More is now understood than they can encompass. The practitioner appreciates that the illness has developed in a particular setting, that it has affected that context, and that others in the social and family field are concerned with and have an impact both on the course of the illness and on its treatment. Yet there are no suitable terms to describe this understanding.

At the same time, it is clear that the onset or exacerbation of an illness galvanizes both the family and the medical systems into action. Certainly, the patient-practitioner relationship is the core of this interaction. And yet it also acts as a hub, drawing other members of both systems into direct contact with the patient and forcing them to deal with questions the illness has raised.

For example, although physicians pocket only 18% of the health care dollar themselves, they control how much of the rest is spent. This is achieved through ordering tests, inviting consultations, sending people to the hospital, prescribing medication, and so on. The medical system depends for its survival on the patients who survive on it for theirs. Without diagnosis, there can be no treatment. Without treatment, there can be no payment. And without payment, nothing moves. The entire medical system hovers in back of the doctor, its outlines barely discerned by the patient's anxious glance, waiting to be triggered into action each time the patient reports a symptom: Will the doctor order X-rays? Will the patient be hospitalized? Will a medication be prescribed? Will a physical therapist be asked to treat the patient? Respiratory therapy? Oxygen? A visiting nurse?

One medical student who sat in our practice for an afternoon asked, "How do you know when to order a CT-scan for someone with a headache? I mean, you don't want to overlook a brain tumor. You could get sued for that, and besides, the patient might be seriously ill and could die." I tried to explain. "You listen to the clinical history. You examine the patient. If it sounds very much like a common headache, you let it ride. If it sounds like a migraine headache, you'll probably try to treat it with the appropriate medications. If the patient's story is funny, or if the presentation doesn't quite ring a bell, or even if the patient and his or her family feel very, very jumpy about the whole thing, then you might want to order a CT-scan. But you can't order a CT-scan on everybody with a headache. Where would all the money come from?"

Where indeed? The medical student was not convinced by my common-sense argument. "But what if, I mean, just suppose, suppose that you made a mistake. And the patient died. You could get sued pretty bad for that, if you didn't order a CT-scan, couldn't you? I mean, couldn't you?"

Of course he was right. That's how millions of dollars get generated by worried doctors through unnecessary X-rays, lab tests, hospitalizations, operations, and so on. The only correct diagnosis here is: defensive behavior by physician in an anxiety-producing situation.

The family and other social groups similarly rely on the physician's activity. After all, the physician's diagnosis makes the patient's illness legitimate. This means the patient can stay home from work. The patient can ask people in the house to bring him or her some hot soup. The patient can take it easy, stay in bed, eat chocolates, watch TV, drink hot tea, and so on. If the doctor had said, "No! You're not sick. Get back to work!" none of this "sickness behavior" would have been possible without a big fight to make it legitimate *in spite of* the physician's reluctance to label it so.

The physician's diagnosis, then, makes the illness legitimate for all those concerned with the patient. Many families will then rearrange themselves to deal with the sickness. Family relationships may shift; someone else may have to take on other caring roles so the family's main caretaker can divert her attention to the patient. This forces a realignment of most family relationships, and creates severe strain in some families. It becomes all right to "take care of" the sick person; it becomes wrong to berate him or her for being weak and/or inactive.

Cultural groups and kinship systems, as well as the social bureaucracies like Disability and Medicaid, will be set into motion by a few diagnostic words from the doctor. "It's his heart, I think it's serious." "I don't think he'll be able to return to work feeling this way; he may be out for as long as three or four weeks." "This woman is unable to work and qualifies for total, permanent disability." "I'm afraid your mother has only a few weeks to live. You should make sure the others in the family know about that and have a chance to see her if they want."

The diagnosis, then, not only is a first step towards organizing the illness, but also organizes the social field surrounding the ill person, which will have to cope with the fact of illness.

As an illness develops, new roles will be determined in the family. Old ones will be relinquished or redefined. Older members of the family weaken and die. Their roles must be taken up by others. Subtle shifts of power and prestige accompany shifts in people's roles, and influence shifts in the meaning structure by which the family develops its values, its appraisal of its own work, and its future goals.

People will move about in response to an illness. A steady parade of visitors passes through the hospital room. Old friends drop in to see the patient who is convalescing. Whole clans assemble when someone is about to die. Wakes assemble an extended social group of friends, family, and acquaintances, and structure people's activity around the care of the bereaved.

Old feuds may emerge or be buried in the heat of illness.

Example 6

Helen and Peggy were twin sisters who had not spoken to one another for three years after a minor argument. But when Helen had to undergo surgery for removal of an ovarian cyst (and possible hysterectomy), Peggy phoned her at the hospital. She "had to set things straight" before the operation. She wanted the two of them to reach an understanding again. Life was too fleeting, too short, too delicately balanced to let petty spats carry on forever.

Illness thus activates and transforms the family system.

Of course, the interrelationship between members of the family and members of the medical system also increases at times of sickness. Family members approach the physician, bearing family secrets or other nuggets of information they feel may be helpful, or else demanding to know why the patient had been allowed to become so ill, whether the illness is catching or hereditary, and what they might do to help out. They ask if the patient can remain at home, if the physician can help find a nursing home bed, if the family can perhaps be given help in getting more money, more care, more social resources.

Family members develop intense relationships with the hospital staff, too. One woman's daughter, for example, developed a profoundly antagonistic relationship with two staff nurses while her mother was ill on their ward. She was convinced the nurses and their colleagues were not providing her mother with the care she needed. Consequently, she carped and criticized, and made herself an extremely unwanted (but frequent) visitor. When it finally became clear to the staff that she was expressing her own frustration about having been unable to care for her mother at home, and was attacking them for the same failure she felt herself, the staff members were able to talk to her kindly about her mother's condition, and help her understand that no one was going to be able to restore the woman to health again, because she was severely sick. This confrontation helped ease the daughter's guilt and led to a great change in her behavior. The nurses now became like close friends to her, for they had "understood" what had been hidden from her understanding for so long and had helped her to see it.

As will be taken up in later sections of this book, illness brings family and patient into contact with a whole range of other social systems: insurance company, courts, workplace, social security, and so on. Often each of these groups has its own physician-expert who, being on salary from the administration, is inclined to take sides with the company (bureaucracy, etc.) against the patient. One result of this is that doctors whose income is derived from different and competing sources often disagree, thereby making the diagnosis of some difficult "cases"—auto accidents, compensation, injuries, suits—a matter only a jury can legally decide.

CHAPTER 6

The Object of Diagnosis:
What Disease Is
Being Diagnosed?

Most people go to the doctor because they don't feel well. They have a problem they can't solve. They don't feel right and don't know why. Patients visit the doctor for a number of reasons, all of which may be "diagnosed" by the clinician. They may have a sore throat, an abscess on a thumb, stitches to be removed. They may simply feel drained and washed out, unduly tired. They may want to obtain drugs, a work-excuse, food stamps, or working papers. They may want birth-control information. They may feel "stuck" in their life and want to talk it over with a physician. They may want to complain about their husband who drinks, their children who are unmanageable and unappreciative, or their mother who is senile and demanding. They may bring a secret to the doctor about another patient. Family physicians (and other primary care physicians) deal with these problems and many more as well.

Usually, patients will begin by talking about a physical problem when they see a doctor. Even if their main reason for coming is to talk about an emotional issue, they may—as we have seen—begin with the physical complaint. Often, too, they may have physical symptoms of some emotional issue, the most obvious example being fatigue and listlessness due to depression. Usually, they expect the physician both to pursue their physical health and to explore other factors which may be involved. (There are exceptions to this, of course: patients who will insist on a

61

physical explanation only, and who will be offended or angry if the physician explores the "mind/body connection." But more about them later.)

Many physicians have gotten into the problem of feeling at ease making a physical diagnosis, but ill at ease making a psychological one. Diagnosis is usually felt to mean a *physical* diagnosis. Other aspects of the patient's problem are put aside, not understood, reserved for the psychiatrist or therapist, and so on. Physicians, upon finding no physical pathology, often feel their job is done, and hasten to "reassure" the patient, who is nevertheless still quite upset by his or her persistent headaches, palpitations, insomnia, chest pains, and the like.

First, however, let us consider the broader question of sickness and disease.

SICKNESS AND DISEASE

Sociologists have tried to distinguish between *sickness* and *disease*. Sickness refers to a person's subjective experience of being ill. Disease refers to the objective pathological condition which is responsible for the symptoms. The physician is asked to diagnose the latter from an evaluation of the patient's complaints, augmented by physical exam and laboratory data. If it were only so simple, there would be no dilemma. The problem is that oftentimes the patient's complaints do not stem from a purely physical condition.

Two figures will help clarify the problem. In the first grid (Figure 7), people are placed into one of four slots, depending on whether they seek medical attention and on whether they have physical signs of illness or not. The grid encompasses everyone.

Positions 1 and 4 pose no problems. People's actions are congruous with the facts. Sick people see the doctor, and healthy people do not. Position 2 includes the "worried well" who often seek medical attention, but are felt to have no significant (physical) disease. And position 3 includes those people who have signs or symptoms of illness but who do not seek medical care.

None of the categories in Figure 7 turn out to be simple. Position 1 depends on agreement of the physicians and their patients about the problem under treatment, or at least agreement about a method of investigating it. If the patient feels she has a physical illness, but the physician feels she does not, and is instead one of the "worried well," the relationship may not last.

Position 4 implies that there is some way of knowing how healthy people are without investigation. But, in effect, almost any patient who comes to the physician is found to have some kind of abnormality, some kind of difficulty. Thus, the "healthy person" is frequently "healthy" only because no physician has been consulted to draw blood, order X-rays, investigate life stresses, and so on, in order to come up with some diagnosis or other. As soon as the healthy person consults the physician, even if only to verify that she is healthy, the situation changes.

Position 2 conceals a great many problems. Some physicians feel that anyone who consults them frequently cannot be "well," although they can indeed be "worried." The category of "somatic fixation" or "somatic obsessional neurosis" has been used to describe this kind of patient, which admittedly forms a very large percentage of the usual physician's office visits. It is no secret that a person's emotional problems can often express themselves in somatic form. If the patient insists on a physical solution, and if the physician finds no physical problems, but only a good deal of situational or characterological stress, bitter wrangling over "the diagnosis" may ensue.

Some examples may illustrate these dilemmas in actual practice.

Example 7

Moving from "worried well" to "sick": Stacey V was a frequent visitor to the physician for a dozen years. She complained of aches in virtually all parts of her body, blurred vision, insomnia, nervousness, palpitations, and a feeling she was going to die. She thought she had some dread disease. Although her symptoms were typical of anxiety, she nevertheless denied she was anxious. Al-

	FINDINGS	NO FINDINGS
FEELING SICK	1	2
FEELING WELL	3	4

Figure 7.

though she had been in marital counseling in the past, she stated everything was going well now. She was simply worried about her physical state. She pleaded for sleeping pills and pep pills. Her husband agreed there was something wrong. The children in the family were all brought to the physician for what seemed to be excessive minor complaints and worry about their health. When one teenage son presented with frank depersonalization, psychiatric consultation was rejected out of hand.

Finally, a laboratory test suggested the possibility of lupus. Stacey became ecstatic. She felt vindicated. She now experienced worsening and remission of her lupus, and insisted that she felt relieved because she had a diagnosis. She read avidly about lupus symptoms. A consultation with a rheumatologist was obtained through a friend. The consultant felt that Stacey most likely did not have lupus, but that, if she did, it was in a very early and mild form, and that her symptoms were "far in excess" of what he imagined her pathological condition warranted.

The family physician felt peeved at the consultation, for it only told him what he already knew, and did not help him move the family from its "somatic fixation" (Huygen and Smits, 1983) to instead focusing on the more pressing and evident emotional/family difficulties.

Example 8

Flora C, a recovered alcoholic, was for 30 years diagnosed as having multiple sclerosis. Her trusted family physician had accomplished this many years previously, on fairly minimal evidence. She attributed everything worrisome in her life to that illness. Whenever work proved too stressful, she had an "attack." When her nerves worsened, she experienced thick speech and staggering gait. When she felt better, these symptoms abated. She continued to live out an "illness" which was not corroborated by any objective proof. She developed a sense of accomplishment at how well she had handled it.

Example 9

Harry D, a 65-year-old married man, was found to have a shadow on his routine chest X-ray, indicative of a large cancer. Though his wife urged him to seek medical attention, he refused repeatedly; he also rejected letters from his physician for follow-up attention. Though objectively ill, he refused to accept the diagnosis.

Example 10

Brenda E, hospitalized for an infection of her leg, was noticed by the nurse to have a large fungating carcinoma of the breast. It had been growing in plain view for more than three years. When asked why she had not sought medical attention, Brenda said she didn't know, but had hoped that the lumps would go away. Despite clear objective signs of "disease," she had managed to deny it to herself.

Other problems with Figure 7 include:

1) Different physicians may interpret data differently, and may ascribe different diseases to the same data.
2) Many people have diseases which are not symptomatic (hypertension, brain tumors).
3) Many illnesses have protean manifestations, and include a large number of "atypical" variants.
4) Many diseases are characterized by physical symptoms which are the same as the symptoms emotional tension—anxiety, excited depression—can produce.
5) Almost everyone has some "problems in living" capable of producing anxiety and worry, which emerge at the least bit of interested questioning.
6) Objective signs of physical illness are frequently not found until the physician looks for them.
7) Hypochondriacs are known to develop "real" disease at some point in their lives.
8) Some worriers are known to be exquisitely sensitive to changes of their internal bodily states, and may actually "perceive" such changes long before the physician's tests can confirm the alteration.

Thus, the discussion of sickness and illness moves to a terrain marked by differences of perspective and opinion, a terrain which has also been explored by sociologists with such guides as the different cultural, class, sexual, and age perspectives of doctor and patient; the different attributions of illness they may make, based on their own particular way of looking at the world; and the different definitions of what constitutes normality.

A further problem is addressed by Figure 8, which portrays the mind/body dichotomy as physicians often conceive it. In circle A, a patient has a physical problem; in circle B, an emotional or mental one.

On Diagnosis

If one returns to Figure 5, it is obvious that a patient can appear physically well, but seem to the physician to have an emotional problem. Or a patient may appear emotionally stable, but have a medical problem. Or he/she may have both—or neither. The "worried well" may be "reframed" as a person with an emotional disorder. The patient who fabricates and pretends to have a physical illness may be redefined as a patient with a serious emotional difficulty. The asthmatic girl who insists, with her family, that the problem is all allergic and infectious, may be dealing directly with the physician on these factors, but may be denying the role of emotional factors, which the physician may see very clearly.

This mind/body dichotomy, then, sets the stage for many arguments, scuffles, and misunderstandings among patients, their families, and physicians. We will return to this in a later section. Suffice it for now to note that this little drawing makes it possible for physicians to "medicalize" everyday life even further, but it also makes it possible to draw back from the overmedicalization of "patients" and see people who come to the physician as having a variety of "problems in living," as Harry Stack Sullivan (1953) so neatly phrased it, some of which may involve medical/physical problems, some of which may involve psychological troubles and emotional suffering, and some of which may involve both.

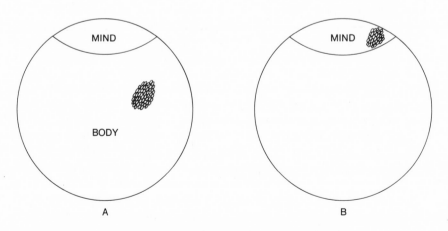

Figure 8. Illness of the mind, illness of the body.

THE MIND/BODY SPLIT PUT TO GOOD USE

The mind/body split underlies much confusion and dissatisfaction in medical practice, on the part of both patient and physician.

The history of psychosomatic medicine has well documented how bodily events affect the mind and vice versa, and has drawn out the constant interplay between emotional and physical factors. And yet, time after time, both patients and physicians act as if "illness" means physical sickness alone, cut off from any relationship with feelings. The growth of *medicine* as the discipline which deals with sickness of the body and *psychotherapy* as that discipline which deals with feeling-states and behavioral problems has kept the mind and the body separated in the therapeutic arena. The public, which learns many of its attitudes from physicians and therapists who sell their skills in the marketplace, has had little choice but to follow the evolving specialization of care. The holistic health movement, accompanied by a strident consumerist rebellion, the women's health movement, and an alternative health movement have all risen in recent years to protest this increased fragmentation of medical care.

In general, problems seen in a medical practice today (especially in a family practice) run the gamut from the almost completely physical to the almost entirely functional. In between are a blend of complex middle-grounds—emotionally induced asthma, irritable stomach related to job stress, pelvic pain linked to sexual difficulties, somatic pains and fear of cancer, and so on. If physicians insist on applying a medical model, they will, of course, emerge with a physical diagnosis all the time. But the more they appreciate problems which involve social or psychological issues, the less satisfied they will be with the purely medical diagnosis.

An integrated approach, which actually begins with the common notion of the split between emotional and physical factors, can help the clinician understand the patient's problem more comprehensively. It can thus serve as an initial way of integrating different factors involved in any patient's presentation, and can extend to looking at a family as well.

This approach attempts to locate the patient's problem on a two-dimensional grid (Figure 9). One axis represents the weight of the perceived psychosocial or emotional aspects of the presenting problem. The other represents the weight of its biomedical aspects. (Different physicians may locate the same patient in different segments of this graph. The same physician, on different days might represent the same patient in different segments. The same patient might "fit" into different segments on different days. All of these are true, but here irrelevant.)

On Diagnosis

Three populations are thus formed: Group 1 consists of problems which appear mainly biological; group 2 consists of "mixed" problems; and group 3 consists of problems which appear mainly psychosocial.

To take examples from the same patient: When she appears in the physician's office with a sore throat, she fits into group 1. When she appears with tension headaches which appear related to squabbles with her husband, she fits into group 2. When she comes in tearful and despondent because the squabbles are getting out of hand, she fits into group 3.

Some physicians may characteristically see all their patients in only one part of the grid. Others may be able to "switch gears" and relate to the different problems at hand.

Such an approach is systemic and pluralistic. It appreciates the range of problems with which patients walk into the physician's office and admits that people change day by day, just as the physician him- or herself changes. Trying to figure out which aspect of the patient's presentation to pursue at any given encounter involves judging what I have referred to as the "brightness" of any given situation or problem.

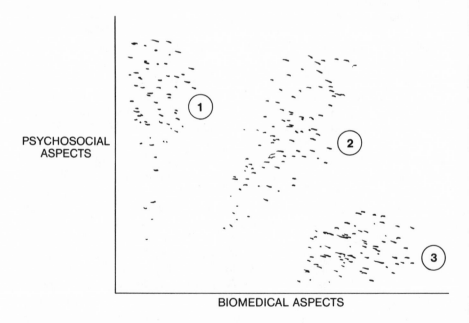

Figure 9. Patients' problems on a grid showing relative weight of psychosocial vs. biomedical issues involved.

IS DIFFICULTY IN LIVING AN ILLNESS?

The physician is always willing, it seems, to extend the definition of illness and come up with a diagnosis for almost any problem. If one accepts the fact that many visits to the physician are occasioned by worry and stress, which produce physical symptoms, then what diagnosis is ascribed to the problem? And what treatment is then to be offered?

The question, raising the demon of "mental illness," brings us back to the mind/body dichotomy.

Unless one claims that all emotional distress is caused by an organic anatomical problem, then using the term "illness" to describe it is metaphorical. When this has been done, it appears to have served humanitarian ends, as when people are granted surcease from responsibility for their own suffering and said to be "sick." But in the medical world, such humanitarianism has an abusive side; and the patient's distress soon becomes transformed into a "disease," thus blurring the real meaning of his or her experience.

This activity also serves to make physicians experts in a wide number of problems which go beyond the confines of medicine. When a patient wishes to talk about marital tension, is that an "illness"? When a woman wonders if she is pregnant, is that an "illness"? When a mother brings in a child and claims he is "hyperactive," is an "illness" involved? Is all of life a medical problem?

Thomas Szasz (1974) has criticized the notion of "mental illness," looking instead at bizarre behavior as *behavior*. He opposes the use of the medical metaphor to redefine moral, legal, social, and personal issues:

> It is impossible to undertake an analysis of the concept of mental illness without first coming to grips with the concept of ordinary or bodily illness. What do we mean when we say that a person is ill? We usually mean two quite different things: first, that he believes, or that his physician believes, or that they both believe, that he suffers from an abnormality or malfunctioning of his body; and second, that he wants, or at least is willing to accept, medical help for his suffering.* The term "illness" thus refers, first, to an abnormal biological condition whose existence may be claimed, truly or falsely, by patient, physician, or others; and second, to the social role of the patient, which may be assumed or assigned.

*Note that in the first case, much conflict may emerge if patient and physician differ. In the second case, conflict may arise over what "medical help" really is.—M.L.G.

> If a person does not suffer from an abnormal biological condition, we do not usually consider him to be ill. . . . And if he does not voluntarily assume the sick role, we do not usually consider him to be a medical patient. [What of patients, hysterical, manipulative, lying, or hypochondriacal, who wish to "assume the sick role" but who are felt to have "no pathology"?] This is because the practice of modern Western medicine rests on two tacit premises—namely, that the physician's task is to diagnose and treat disorders of the human body, and that he can carry out these services only with the consent of his patient. In other words, physicians are trained to treat bodily ills—not economic, moral, racial, religious, or political "ills." . . . Strictly speaking, then, disease or illness can affect only the body. Hence, there can be no such thing as mental illness. The term . . . is a metaphor. (pp. viii-ix)

Alas, physicians today are trained to treat emotional problems as well. And, willy-nilly, whatever problems physicians treat must be defined as "illnesses" because 1) operationally, physicians treat illness, and 2) physicians cannot be reimbursed for their work unless it is characterized as treatment of an illness. From this dilemma arises the objections of Illich (1976) and others concerned with the creeping "medicalization of everyday life."

The advances of the medical model have provided psychiatric terms for all of medicine. There is a term available for every difficulty—stress reaction of adolescence, reactive depression, psychophysiological gastrointestinal disturbance. Admittedly, these are all "individual" terms. But, would the development of even family-oriented diagnostic categories help save patients and their families from being devoured and defined by the medical model of distress? Would this be advisable?

Example 11

Joanne F comes to the office, voice aquiver and hands trembling. She has been fighting with her son. She cannot breathe. She is afraid she has heart trouble, cancer, whatever. She is divorced, and has had trouble holding a job. Her boss criticizes her work. She is underpaid. She has no time for her son and is worried about him.

What does it mean, to write on a diagnostic slip "palpitations," or "anxiety reaction," or even "anxiety reaction in a single mother"?

Two tendencies struggle for dominance in family practice today. One insists that emotional problems are indeed "illnesses," but says they belong in the domain of the mental health professional. The other agrees that emotional problems are "illnesses" but insists that the family doctor can treat them. A third position, that the emotional problems people experience are *not* "illnesses," even though they may provoke physical distress which brings people to the physician, and even though they may in fact lead to actual physical disturbance (ulcers, heart attacks), has not found many advocates. Yet this seems obviously true to me.

Family physicians have a role in helping patients "work out" their problems in living, some of which may be associated with physical distress. The tendency to have to give diagnoses for this work arises from the market conditions and professional role of the physician.

IS THE DIAGNOSED ILLNESS THE PATIENT'S PROBLEM?

Traditional medicine spends much effort seeking a physical diagnosis, which it can then treat as fact. This orientation comes from many factors, not the least of which is the patient's principally announced reason for coming to the doctor: an ailment of the body.

Patients expect the physician to be an expert in ills of the body. They do not expect the primary-care doctor to be a minister, a lawyer, or a psychotherapist. Nor do most physicians today behave differently. They doggedly pursue the physical, virtually to the exclusion of everything else. In a way, it is as if most physicians have automatically heard Szasz's warnings about medicine's tendency to reach into every area of life (where it doesn't belong), and make expert pronouncements. So they, like their patients, usually tend to emphasize the physical.

What is the problem, then? The problem is that many problems of the body are intimately related to problems in the mind, to feeling-states, chronic strain and stress, and the effects on the body of humors and hormones affected by emotional stress and mediated through the corticosteroids, epinephrine, norepinephrine, and the nervous system. If patients do not expect an integrated approach from their physician, and if they do not accept such an approach when they find it, they will not be able to find relief from the suffering which brought them to the office in the first place.

Some patients, for example, are troubled by physical ailments, and do not recognize their link to stress. Others know full well that something else is worrying them, but are unable to speak directly to the physician about it, so they use the physical ailment as a "ticket" to gain access to the doctor's time.

The physician's emphasis on physical diagnostics, grounded in his own training, in what he thinks the patient is asking for, and in the financial incentives which structure most medical practice, leads to an exaggerated concern with blood tests, X-rays, and other more expensive and more risky technical procedures. This is what Balint described as "eliminating by appropriate physical examinations." Only if no "organic" illness is found, after a series of exhaustive examinations and tests, biopsies, consultations, and so on, will the physician be prepared to grant that the illness may be stress-related or psychosomatic. (Of course, at such a time, the patient may be helplessly referred on to the psychotherapist with a note from the physician stating that she is "in good physical health: no pathology found.")

There is such a ubiquitous fear of "missing something" in medicine that the physician will order a dozen unnecessary tests to avoid overlooking a serious physical illness ("I could get sued!"). On the other hand, the most obvious anxiety state or depressive symptom may go untreated and virtually unmentioned and unexplored . . . for months!

As Balint points out, there is also a danger, "not only in missing a physical sign, but also in finding one." The patient suffers from dyspepsia and cramps. A set of X-rays is performed, and the patient is found to have gallstones. Now the physician and the patient have a problem: clear physical evidence has been uncovered which is "consistent" to some degree with the patient's symptoms. Should an operation be performed? Often, such a procedure is indeed performed. The symptoms abate for three months. And then they return. The pain was not due to gallstones after all. But now the patient may be developing pain from intestinal adhesions, etc., etc.

A modest hiatal hernia may be found on X-ray. Antacids and diet are duly prescribed. But epigastric pain and burning persist. At this point, the patient and physician usually come to some kind of squabble. The patient, who has agreed with the physical diagnosis, complains that "I'm not getting any better!" and implies that the physician doesn't know what he's talking about. The physician complains that the patient isn't following instructions, or—sensing that the physical diagnosis isn't the whole story—may at this point begin suggesting that part of the problem may be stress-related. At this point the patient may complain bitterly, "So you think it's all in my head, do you!" and redouble her criticisms of the doctor's diagnostic acumen.

Some physicians have suggested working at both levels—physical and emotional—from the beginning. Certainly, this makes sense, especially since four weeks of physical tests without a hint that the problem may be more-than-physical may very well convince the patient that the problem is indeed basically physical, that the physician thinks this, too, and is thereby ordering the vast array of tests, and so on. For the physician to switch perspective later may seem a sign of failure, and may both diminish the patient's confidence in the physician and increase her resistance to dealing with the psychosocial context of her suffering.

But working both levels from the start may be hard to do, particularly if the symptoms could be due to some simply treatable, easily diagnosed illness: Why then open the whole bag of worms about the patient's emotional life, thereby implying that there's some kind of problem, when the patient feels the main thing is a physical abnormality which the physician had damn well better find and treat—period.

Rather than probing the illness more broadly, most physicians are thus content to narrow it down, pin a physical name on it, and deal with it. The usual consultation provides an excellent example of this mentality. If nothing orthopedic is found, the report comes back "no orthopedic pathology," and the consultant's task is finished. Physicians and patients are thus both reinforced in viewing bodily distress in terms of some fundamentally physical dysfunction.

A further problem is that *all patients have psychosocial problems*. Everyone's life is in flux, under stress, forced to change and adapt. In addition, many patients may have more than one problem, more than one illness. People must all deal with making a living, paying the rent, buying food, raising their kids, getting along with their families, staying on reasonable terms with their neighbors, and so on. People must cope with their own inner feelings, which are constantly being pummelled and altered by social relationships and by life changes. Worries over one's worth, one's identity, the value of one's work, the safety of one's intimates, and so on create a constantly agitated "internal milieu." These heaped-up social and psychological factors form a honeycomb in which each of us lives. When physical woes and physical illness are added to this picture, the effect can be troublesome, cataclysmic, devastating.

On top of this, different physical ailments form a matrix of their own, abetted by whatever forms of treatment have been prescribed for them. Thus, the patient with renal failure may develop salt and fluid imbalance. The patient with arthritis may develop side-effects of the anti-inflammatory medications given, which may mimic (or even lead to) ulcer disease. If heart disease is present as well, the two diseased systems interact, possibly with increased ill effect; and medication prescribed for one condition may adversely affect the other. Physical ailments and their treatment may thus create cascades of newer, more worrisome ills. The weary patient with congestive heart failure may be made even more tired by the Capoten or Inderal the physician prescribes. The patient with hypertension may experience painful calf cramps because of diuretic-induced potassium depletion. Patients, of course, do not sort out all these different effects. They are only aware of "feeling worse," "aching all over," and so on.

Given this exceedingly complicated matrix, the physician is supposed to sift through the various elements which may be contributing to the problem and figure out what is "really" bothering the patient. The patient, to be sure, may have a different idea of this (such dilemmas will be considered in Section II), and may pursue a different agenda entirely.

To sum this up, the patient comes to the physician with a set of complaints which may be mainly physical, emotional, or both. Both patient and physician have their own agenda, their own perspectives. Furthermore, each lives in a psychosocial context fraught with conflict and change. The patient may have a number of physical or psychological ailments, and may be taking medications which further affect his or her physical and mental state. *Diagnoses are additive and interactive.* It takes an astute clinician to focus on one particular set of "causes" for the complaints the patient most wishes to present, and to know at the same time how to probe for complaints which seem "just beneath the surface" and which the patient will acknowledge after questioning but not spontaneously volunteer.

THE OBJECT OF DIAGNOSIS IN FAMILY PRACTICE

I sometimes feel that my patients' physical complaints, which I am (successfully) treating, are all the same superficial to their lives. They continue to grapple with problems which create far more distress than the things I am treating. What is appropriate to family practice? How much should the physician probe? How much is supposed to fit into the physician-patient relationship? Should family conferences be called, even when the patient does not want it?

Approximately 75% of the patients who cross the family physician's threshold bring significant psychosocial issues. As physicians come to know patients and their families, and as they come to understand themselves well enough to trust their reactions to patients in any given situation, they learn to deepen their sense of the harmony between the physical and emotional factors at work. Part of the clinician's skill, therefore, is knowing when to pursue one avenue, and when to pursue another. The patient may come in announcing one problem, but this has to be seen as merely the opening move in a rather lengthy process of negotiating the disease. The second move is up to the physician.

In family practice the problem is complicated by patients' coming in on other days as caretakers, parents, children, concerned friends, and so on. They come in for different problems on different days:

> A mother is upset because her teenage daughter is getting drunk and running around with older boys; on her follow-up visit for a vaginal infection, she requests a sedative but is hesitant to talk further about the daughter's problem. Instead, she wants the physician to confront the girl on her next visit.

> A worker comes in with back pains, afraid he may become disabled. The next week, his child comes in for a camp physical. The mother seems clearly worried, but will not talk in the child's presence, and she is in a hurry to get back home.

Each day has a constant mix of problems. Psychosocial woes mingle with physical ones, sometimes following one upon the next, sometimes intertwined. A woman who cannot afford medicine comes in with recurrent infection. A teenage girl is pregnant and has decided against an abortion; she presents now with a bad cough. A man comes in to get some sutures taken out. An elderly couple comes in for their monthly blood pressure check and renewal of medications. A paranoid woman comes in complaining that someone is trying to poison her, and announces that she has terminated her homemaker because she was part of the general plot against her. A depressed elderly woman comes in with chest pains, and asks for pills to help her lose weight.

> Even when they do fall under medical categories, the patients' illnesses may not be the precipitating cause of their visit. The illness may be an excuse to see the physician in hopes he will address what is "really" bothering them. A similar mechanism may lead a woman to bring her "sick" child into the office and then comment, just as she is leaving, "Oh, by the way, doc, I been wondering. Harry's been . . ."

Considering the number of illnesses felt to be brought about or aggravated by stress, the number of illnesses which are used as "tickets" to the doctor's office, and the number of admittedly psychological problems that patients present to their doctor, then the figure of 75% of family practice visits having a significant psychosocial component becomes better understood. How then does the focus on diagnosis as a physical problem jibe with this?

Clearly, part of the promise of family practice lies in finding a better way of describing the balance of physical and psychosocial factors that bring patients to the physician's office, and in helping reformulate the patient-practitioner relationship.

CHAPTER 7

The Content of Diagnosis: Fact or Hypothesis?

DIAGNOSIS AS A HYPOTHESIS

The origin of the word suggests that diagnosis is an act which leads to some form of knowledge, that it corresponds to some external reality, some verifiable fact, some truth. Certainly, this is how traditional medicine views diagnosis: as a statement of fact. According to this traditional model, the astute clinician, reflecting on the particular concatenation of physical findings, subjective complaints, blood and X-ray reports, etc., in the light of his or her past experience and knowledge of the medical literature, thus arrives at the "truth" of the patient's disease.

This knowledge then structures rational treatment of the disease, aimed at easing the patient's suffering and curing the malady.

But is this notion accurate? In what way is diagnosis a *fact*, rather, say, than a conjecture or an educated guess? And what would it mean to say that a diagnosis is "true" or "correct"?

A diagnosis emerges as a conclusion, an opinion. Whether it is "true" depends on several criteria: Does the patient's illness follow the course predicted by that diagnosis? Is it at least consistent with it? Does treatment aimed at the diagnosed illness cure the patient's problem? Can any other possible diagnosis fit the same observed facts and reported symptoms?

Even these criteria are not absolute. For example, the patient's sickness may be self-limited and scheduled to improve no matter what is done, even when the physician's diagnosis is wrong—as when the doctor, diagnosing bacterial pharyngitis, prescribes penicillin, and the patient improves because the problem was only a viral infection in the first place. Or, to take another example, it may be that several different disease processes are possible—in dermatology, for example—but the empirical treatment for them all is the same: steroids. In this latter instance, the patient will get well whether the physician has made the correct diagnosis—the one which a biopsy would prove, under the microscope—or not.

In fact, the more closely one looks, the more it appears that—except in a limited number of cases, such as broken bones, hemorrhoids, strep throat, and the like—diagnosis is always more an educated guess than a certainty. After all, how far do physicians have to pursue a microscopic or laboratory proof of each of their diagnoses? Does every headache demand a CT-scan to "rule out" a brain tumor? Does every episode of indigestion require an upper GI series? Does every incidence of shoulder pain warrant EMG's, X-rays, etc.? Practitioners usually obtain tests when they feel they need more data in order to provide treatment. If the diagnosis appears fairly obvious, the clinician tries *treating* it, not doing a dozen tests. In addition, as has become very clear recently, financial considerations are involved, too, which makes treating patients different from working in a lab.

Yet the problem continues on other levels. Even when it comes to something "easy," like a bleeding ulcer, more questions can be asked: What caused the ulcer? Is it malignant or benign? Is it related to aspirin use? Is it related to stress? How exactly did stress manage to "cause" the ulcer? Is the patient genetically predisposed to develop ulcer disease? Are other dietary factors involved? The questions are not trivial. Each of them is related to subsequent management and advice.

Diagnosis, like any other scientific hypothesis, is a conjecture, whose purpose is to explain the ailing patient's symptoms in the hopes of alleviating them. A hypothesis is not a statement of fact. It is "an unproved theory, proposition, supposition, etc. tentatively accepted to explain certain facts or to provide the basis for further investigation" (Webster's Unabridged Dictionary). It can be discarded if subsequent experience indicates that it is wrong or incomplete. It can be amended, reworked, corrected. A diagnosis, in other words, is an evolving, live entity which is used to guide practice.

In this sense, a hypothesis is a hunch or supposition, which follows a *probabilistic*, not a *mechanistic*, paradigm (Bursztajn et al., 1981). According to this paradigm, causality is not a strictly linear concept, but a notion more in line with contemporary ideas of randomness and uncertainty, and with the movements in scientific thought which have characterized 20th century physics. Certainty and linear causality are oddities "at one end of the curve," reserved for the simpler medical problems.

QUESTIONS OF CERTAINTY AND UNCERTAINTY

Bursztajn and his co-workers (1981) have argued that medical decisions rest on weighing one set of probabilities against another. Treatment is steeped in uncertainty. One treatment may have more potential complications than another, but offers a higher chance for cure. Another treatment is simpler and less noxious, but it is possibly less effective: Which does the patient do first? When the physician wants to diagnose the problem, how far will the patient permit him or her to go? Does everyone who survives a heart attack need coronary angiography? Does everyone with dizziness need carotid arteriograms? How much risk is acceptable for a diagnostic procedure? How much new knowledge can be gained? What difference will it make in the treatment? How much uncertainty can the patient and his or her family tolerate?

Example 12

Sam D had been troubled with the complications of arteriosclerosis. Six years ago he had gone through a heart attack. He was currently on medication for angina. Two years ago he had gone to a vascular surgeon because his leg throbbed when he walked. The surgeon, after taking tests of his circulation, including arteriograms, had advised an arterial bypass graft, saying that the circulation in the main artery to the leg was badly compromised by thick fatty plaques. Sam has gone through the procedure.

Now he had experienced numbness of the left and right arm, more so on the left. He went back to the vascular surgeon, who, after doing tests, suggested that the main arteries to his head were narrowing, and that he might need surgery again. Sam then went to his family physician, who agreed that a workup might be helpful, but advised caution until this was completed.

Hospitalization took place. The vascular surgeon ordered arter-

iograms, which showed some moderate plaque formation in the
carotid artery on the left, but no real impairment of flow. A neurologist was called in. He argued that Sam's symptoms did not fit
the supposed lesion, and said the surgery would not be aimed at
the symptoms, which he felt came from arthritis of the spine. An
internist was called in, too, especially in view of Sam's past heart
attack. He agreed with the neurologist. So did the family doctor.
"Sam," he said, "there's really no indication that the problem they
find on the arteriogram is causing the numbness. And the operation
does carry risks."

In the meantime, however, the surgeon had told Sam that the
findings suggested he was in danger of a stroke at any time. "If
a piece of that plaque breaks off, you could have a stroke." He
advised Sam to have a "prophylactic" endarterectomy anyway, to
ward off future chances of such a complication.

Sam decided to have the operation. "Doc," he said, "I know it
won't help the numbness. But how can I go to sleep at night,
thinking that any minute I might get a stroke, die, who knows
what. . . ?" The surgeon had frightened him, and he now insisted
on having the procedure done. The surgeon felt it was the correct
decision, even though it was now based on a different set of reasons.

If this web of uncertainty surrounds decisions involving treatment,
it also surrounds decisions concerning the initial diagnosis. Given a
limited amount of data—for neither the patient's body nor his checkbook
can afford indefinite testing—the physician must reach some sort of
working diagnosis. If he and the patient, following Balint's description,
agree on it, then they will move ahead to treatment, and change the
original diagnosis only if treatment fails, if symptoms worsen, or if some
other, newer information emerges.

Before we go further, let us clarify exactly what it is we are trying to
diagnose. The traditional view assumes that all illness can be traced back
to abnormalities of one of two types—problems of morbid structure or
anatomy (ulcers, tumors, infections) and problems of morbid function
or physiology (overactive thyroid, weakened heart, abnormal immune
response). The two are, of course, interlinked. But the medical advances
of the early 19th century emphasized the former, while the late 19th and
early 20th century emphasized the latter.

Both focus on physical illness, of course, and only serve to deepen
the mind/body split. Whatever the patient's symptoms, the physician
struggles to find the physical cause, whether in a deranged anatomy or

a malfunctioning physiology. There is no place in such a system for contextual medicine. There is simply no point of entry, no intersection.

If this kind of *physical* diagnosis is sought, then it carries its own measure of uncertainty with it. These are addressed by Engle and Davis (1963), by Feinstein (1967), and by others who probe the ambiguities of physical diagnosis. But if a different, more integrated kind of diagnosis is sought, one which rests on seeing the patient's problems along the grid suggested in the last chapter, where both biomedical and psycho-social/emotional factors are involved, then our very notion of "disease" has to change; we must find terms for identifying the context, the feel, the setting, the use, the interpersonal dynamics, and the internal meaning of the sickness, as well as whatever physical abnormality may exist. Such a nosology does not yet exist.

ENGLE AND DAVIS: DIFFERENT ORDERS OF CERTAINTY

To be fair about it, Engle and Davis' "five orders of certainty" (1963, see p. 8) correspond to most clinicians' experience. Some physical problems are simple to diagnose; others, more complex. The more embedded in murky psychosomatic process, the more sticky is the task of diagnosis. The more complicated the physiological or biochemical processes involved, the more difficult it is to find "the" explanation.

The following has been developed from Engle and Davis' initial categorization, but I have taken a good deal of liberty with it, in an attempt to bring it more up to date, in line with problems more clinicians are familiar with facing:

1) The first order of certainty represents well-defined ailments whose etiological agent is both clear and simple, and whose disease picture is fairly characteristic. This is the case with fractured bones, acute infections, burns and frostbite, congenital infections, and many cancers.
2) The second order of certainty represents easily diagnosed diseases whose causes may be numerous, interactive, or yet unclear. Such is the case with diabetes, hypertension, ulcers, and some forms of auto-immune diseases, as well as the different degenerative diseases.
3) The third order of certainty represents illnesses with an evident emotional or functional component, as well as primarily emotional disorders. The "cause" again appears murky or multitudinous. This is the case, for example, with acute depressive reactions, chronic

irritable bowel syndrome, neurodermatitis, allergic disorders, asthma, and the like.

4) A fourth order of certainty involves processes open to conjecture, whose clinical picture is not fully explicable, but which represent recognizable entities all the same. Examples of this include the various syndromes medicine has established, as well as a large number of descriptive syndromes which essentially represent problems in living: stress reactions, marital discord, adolescent adjustment reactions, life-stage problems. Each of these may, of course, have physical as well as emotional components.

5) The fifth order of certainty involves ailments which present themselves to the physician in a baffling, overdetermined, and complex fashion, seeming to involve functional as well as physical factors at a number of different levels. Such problems are exceedingly difficult to unravel. For example, an elderly woman with chronic heart disease, chronic bowel trouble, and chronic depression appears with a worsening of her abdominal complaints, in a context of having heard that her oldest son has just been admitted to an intensive care unit with a heart attack. Diagnosing her "problem" involves many determinants at once. A good number of presentations among the elderly, neurotic and psychophysiological reactions, functional aches and pains, depressive equivalents, and so on all fall into this category at some time or another.

Faced with an ever-increasing tangle of stress-related, genetic, environmental, biochemical, immunological, etc. factors, the clinician may be impelled to move ever more to notions resembling those which family therapists are finding useful: notions of "fit" and "coherence" (Dell and Goolishian, 1979). The closer an illness is to the traditional model of disease, the more likely it is to be capable of simple proof, to be diagnosed with a high degree of certainty. Massive coronaries, broken bones, nosebleeds: These are simple. Continued epigastric distress in the face of a "normal" upper GI series presents a problem.

Questions of uncertainty in diagnosis can emerge at many different levels:

• *Host resistance, timing.* A simple and easily diagnosed problem, like strep throat, raises questions about why this particular child contracted this particular disease, now. In the case of a simple broken bone, questions can be raised about motivation, for example, about whether the patient is "accident-prone," or whether emotional worry and preoccupation led to lessened surveillance on the patient's part.

- *Multiple possible explanations.* Problems may admit of several different solutions—like a headache, which can be caused by elevated blood pressure, eye strain, tension, or brain tumor. Thus, they always have built-in uncertainty. A woman with benign fibrocystic disease of the breast, for example, may develop a breast cancer at any time, but to the clinician there may appear to be no change in the lumpiness of the two breasts. How often is a mammogram necessary? How often is a mammogram wrong? How large does a tumor have to be to be diagnosed with 90% certainty by mammography? One pursues a limited set of possibilities, always with the understanding that error is possible.
- *Sampling error, lab error.* Problems may arise with lab tests and X-rays. They may be wrong. There may be other causes of "positive" findings than the one disease in question—such as a falsely positive VDRL, or a positive ANA which is caused by some viral problem, not by a collagen disease. Procedures of collecting the specimen may be faulty: The urine may sit around and become "contaminated." Stool may no longer be "fresh" when it is examined, and the parasites will no longer be visible.
- *Problems of causality, mind/body linkages.* Take a patient with an ulcer. What is the role of psychosomatic factors—what "caused" the ulcer? Or, in the case of abdominal pain, where no physical abnormality is found and where the pain is attributed to "emotional" factors (common in children), how does emotional stress "cause" the abdominal pain?
- *Other mind/body problems.* Why is a depressed person losing weight—might it be cancer as well as depression? If anxiety causes palpitations, what is the best way of treating it? What about the side-effects of medications? What about the placebo effect?

The list could be extended for some length. Whatever answers can be given at one level engender further questions at another.

In practice, treatment and diagnosis are part of the same coin (Brody and Waters, 1980). One intervenes therapeutically, going by the clinical impression. The patient's subsequent response to treatment can give important information which affects the original diagnosis. Failure of treatment usually implies an erroneous initial impression (or non-compliance, faulty technique, drug-resistance, and so on).

A CONTEXTUAL APPROACH NEEDED FOR
COMPLEX DIAGNOSTIC PROBLEMS

To return to Figure 7 (in Chapter 6), problems which fit into positions 1 and 4 can be simply treated. But problems which mix psychosocial and biomedical factors need a contextual approach. The biomedical model, which holds little place for contextual factors, family dynamics, or multifactorial etiology, has trouble coping with the 50-80% of routine office visits to a busy family physician, in which physical complaints float amidst a sea of everyday psychosocial problems.

Even the simplest of illnesses, easily "diagnosed" by biomedical criteria, becomes a mass of unclarity when the illness is placed in its family context. Is the illness disabling? Is the patient complying with treatment; if not, why not? Are others in the family likely to come down with the same illness? Has the truth about the diagnosis been told; if so, to whom? Diagnosis is often but a prelude to the task of managing the patient and the illness. In this sense, nothing, not even the simplest strep throat, is an easy matter for the physician. Further dilemmas based on other systemic levels—cellular, immunological, family, workplace, school—are likely to emerge.

If the biomedical model has problems even when it comes to simple causes of illness, it has even greater difficulty in dealing with interrelated or simultaneous causative factors. It flounders when it tries to explain the differing expressions of illness and cannot adequately deal with psychological issues (except to make a diagnosis of mental illness) or with uncertainty.

Example 13

Barbara G comes to the physician for an initial visit. She has horrible headaches. Her heart pounds. Her fingers are numb and tingling. In addition, her stomach is in knots. She has pains when she urinates, and a vaginal discharge. She is afraid of a nervous breakdown.

On further questioning, she says her husband died three years ago. She is worried about her 12-year-old daughter who is entering adolescence. She is on welfare, but she is trying to get off. Her mother has been sick.

Initial appraisal is made, which includes the strong likelihood of anxiety attacks in a woman facing critical life stresses. In addition, she appears to have both a urinary tract infection and vaginitis, reflecting a probable lowered resistance to disease.

Treatment is a combination of antibiotic medication and mild sedatives, given in a supportive context which understands the psychosocial pressures she is experiencing, and also raises the question of future counseling.

QUESTIONS OF BREADTH AND DEPTH

We have seen that a diagnosis can be made at a number of different levels, and with a wider or more narrow scope. Each of these corresponds to a different way of viewing illness, a different conception of diagnosis, and a different view of the doctor's function.

One definition of depth and breadth comes from G. Gayle Stephens (1982). He describes *breadth* as "the universal interest," thus suggesting its overall scope, and *depth* as "the historical perspective," thus suggesting an appreciation of the evolution of something over time. Something more, though, seems to be involved in what we commonly mean by these terms.

Breadth of diagnosis reflects the expanse of scope we apply to a matter at hand. This can even include an appreciation of historical data as well. Our sense of depth involves often-hidden meanings and our attributions of experience: psychological feelings, memories, recollections, fears and dreams, anxieties, recapitulations of past experiences in our present-day life, values, beliefs, assumptions.

Pursuing the sense of breadth, one can diagnose: the various physical ailments; the body's response to the illness at various organ system and cellular levels; the patient's personality structure; the precipitating environmental and situational problems; the social context which harbors the development and appearance of the illness; the type of family structure and family stress being experienced; and so on. Although practicing physicians usually find that this broader, more comprehensive diagnosis expresses more fully what they want to know, they may on occasion "stick with" a simpler and less comprehensive level. Not every encounter has to be "grand passion." Questions of depth, on the other hand, usually involve psychological perception and insight.

The simplest (narrowest) model of disease stems from a linear view and is the most basic level of physical diagnosis: "Yep, it's a strep throat, John." Or, "Well, it looks like you've got real bad circulation here." The patient is usually satisfied with this level of diagnosis, if his or her presenting complaints have been caused by that problem, if the problem can be eased or cured, and if treatment will result in rapid amelioration of the suffering.

The next expanse of diagnosis is the multifactor explanation. The patient has a genetic predisposition to develop the sickness. A viral illness predisposes to its appearance. The infection adversely affects the patient's immune system, and the illness then ensues—let us say, the beginnings of rheumatoid arthritis. Stress factors, related to work or marital factors, loss, and so on can further impair the competence of the immune system to cope with offending factors, thus increasing the chance that illness will occur.

This type of explanation accepts a variety of factors and begins to explore some of the factors of chance and probability that lead to one person's falling ill while another, seemingly exposed to the same agents and stresses, remains well. [For a further discussion of the role of stress and illness, see Cannon (1920), Selye (1956), Locke (1982), Ader (1982), Lipowski et al. (1977).]

The systemic expanse, which sees "systems in interaction" as part of a kinetic, shifting world, is perhaps the furthest category of broad diagnosis. Here, the physician is cognizant of factors as disparate as the environment, work-related hazards and toxins, the role of recent loss and worry, exposure to illness, genetic makeup, and so on. More importantly, the physician is also aware of the interrelatedness of these factors, seeing them as each affecting one another, not as separate etiological agents, whose effects are somehow "summed up" through the illness. This conception, essentially a conception of causality, has been expressed through a simple drawing by Christie-Seely (1981) (Figure 10).

The notion of depth appears close to what Balint (1957) was talking about with his "deeper level of diagnosis," which views patients in their psychosocial life context. It also includes much that has been learned through interest in communication and interaction, such as the work on attributions by Waitzkin and Stoeckle (1976), which highlights how patient and physician may perceive the illness in quite different and mutually contradictory ways.

How does this come out in practice? One way certainly is around the diagnostic code written down for the patient's illness—that is, around nosology.

Rather than writing down that a patient has "headache," we might be more interested in characterizing a number of things. For example, we might conceive of a diagnosis as reflecting:

1) The physical problem(s).
2) The patient's psychosocial and life-stage situation.
3) The role of the patient's family dynamics or life-stage problem.

4) The role of other natural or social systems—workplace, environment, genetic, generational, church group, neighborhood, etc.
5) The illness's meaning in its personal, family, cultural, etc. contexts.

Thus, the person with a headache might obtain a broader and deeper diagnosis, which comments on a "tension headache in an obsessional, depressed, somewhat isolated 30-year-old married man afraid of losing his job, and worrying about money." Or one might diagnose, "irritable stomach syndrome with epigastric burning, in a masochistic, passive single woman who finds it difficult to discuss her feelings, and who is still tied to her parents."

Certainly, the broader and deeper one goes, the less succinct becomes the diagnosis. And, for many uses, a brief biomedical diagnosis is more than adequate, especially in view of threats to the confidentiality of information these days. But, for proper payment-for-services-rendered, it will be necessary to develop diagnostic codes and terms which relate

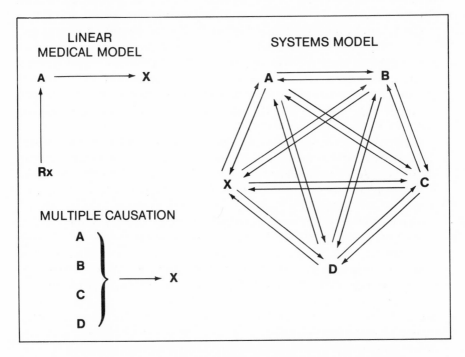

Figure 10. Three causality schemes (after Christie-Seely, 1981).

to family and social issues, so that the physician will not have to define his or her work as only treating physical illness.

Unless the broader dimensions of medical (family) practice are recognized by including social and family diagnostic codes and terms, as well as the individual ones, it will be impossible to advance and expand family practice. Payment will be lacking. And research, which depends on the accumulation of data, will be hampered because if family codes, terms, etc., are not available, each researcher will have to invent his or her own terms, squabbling will ensue, etc., etc.

For this reason, efforts such as Lee Hyde's (unpublished manuscript, 1984), in trying to arrive at a nosology which embraces family and social problems, as well as problems familiar to physical medicine, are critically important. So are, I might add, the increased use of genograms, family trees, family charts, draw-a-circle pictures, and so on, in the charts of family practitioners, for they increase the data base of family and social factors involved in the patient's presentation.

One need hardly point out that this view of diagnosis and nosology is not now being taught in the medical schools. Yet it is a view which fits the experience of most primary-care practitioners.

Carmichael and Carmichael (1981) have commented that approximately 80% of the encounters with the family physician follow a "relational model" which is "not concerned with cure or control of disease but rather with the attention, support, and comfort the patient receives" (p. 126). Despite other studies which emphasize the biomedical content of family practice (Rosenblatt et al., 1982), our own experience agrees with the Carmichaels' view.

Any busy day is filled with a variety of problems. A mother comes in upset because her teenage son is using drugs, and asks for a sedative for herself. A factory worker comes in with shoulder pains and wonders if the problem is work-related and if he should return to work or stay home. A girl comes in with pain in the belly and a negative exam. A woman comes in with a sore throat, and says she needs a family doctor. A man comes in asking for drugs, and seems to be addicted. A teenage girl comes in with abdominal pain; she is pregnant, unbeknownst to her mother (Is there an obligation to tell, if the patient insists she does not want anyone told?) and has decided to keep the child. A 23-year-old man comes in for removal of sutures. A harried secretary comes in for a blood pressure check, and complains about how she is being treated at work. A woman on welfare comes in to complain about the forced work program, which has made her sit in the middle of an office of gaping men, who use her to go for their coffee and errands, all at a minimum wage. An elderly couple comes by for an every-three-month checkup, medication refill, and blood tests; they bring in the latest pictures of their grandchildren and stories of Christmas. A depressed woman comes in complaining that she cannot lose weight and that her back hurts. A lonely widow complains that her arthritis is killing her, and that no one in her family cares about her anymore. A 50-year-old man comes in, worried that his medication might be making him impotent. And on and on.

What diagnostic terms can be given to describe these transactions? When the encounter is done, what few and simple words, what set of prearranged digits should the physician scrawl down on the "encounter form" to explain the illness, the reason for the patient's having come in the first place?

It is simplest of all to write down "hypertension" or "low back pain." It is even fetching to write down "anxiety attack" or "irritable bowel syndrome." There is as yet no adequate nosology which describes the experience of family practice (although Lee Hyde is working at it). Even if such a nosology existed, however, would it do justice to the complexity of the encounter? Would physicians then have to check off three, four, five, or more different categories for each visit? Would this make up the "broad" diagnostic picture? Would it be available via computer banks to any prying eye? What about the confidentiality and privacy of the patient? Some psychotherapists are known to keep two sets of records: their own and the "official" book. Would family physicians have to begin doing the same thing? What would happen if the patient found out the "real" diagnosis?

Insurance companies do not recognize family-based diagnoses. Should they? Would remuneration for dealing with problems occasioned by family stress help family medicine develop, or would it herald the field's demise?

Diagnosis is not an end in itself. It is always a "working hypothesis," a way of viewing the patient as a whole. This view needs to be taught to medical students, starting on the very first day they enter school.

Example 14

Walter H appears at the office with an asthma attack. He is also drunk, the first time the physician has seen him this way in three years. His wife and two of his three children are with him. As it turns out, his eldest son has just been arrested and is now in jail. Worry led him to drink heavily, and now he has developed an

asthma attack. The family is very worried. Treatment is indeed in
the realm of family practice: What is the diagnosis?

DIAGNOSIS AS A WORKING HYPOTHESIS

The content of a diagnosis reflects the clinician's goals in making it.
Its certainty as a statement of fact varies according to how closely it fits
traditional patterns of disease. Its descriptive content varies with the
depth and breadth of the physician's outlook.

For the majority of medical complaints, a diagnosis is a working hypothesis, which admits varying degrees of uncertainty. It is a useful
guide to treatment. Having such a hypothesis lessens both the patient's
and the physician's anxiety levels and permits them to move on to the
next stage of dealing with the disease in its proper context.

Bursztajn's probabilistic paradigm is important to this process. Not
only is uncertainty built into every diagnosis, but it is also built into all
forms of treatment. Treatment affects diagnosis; diagnosis orients treatment. A dialectical theory of knowledge is thus put into practice, with
each stage of intervention giving more information about the process at
hand, and each deepened understanding leading to better intervention.
The diagnosis expresses the level of understanding about the process
which has been reached at any given time. Looked at in this way, nothing
is permanent or inflexible about any diagnostic impression. Every diagnosis must be tested in practice and over time. Errors are inevitable,
but can be minimized by astute clinical skill and judgment.

CHAPTER 8

Conclusion: A Practical Approach to Diagnosis

A theory may be elegant but useless if it cannot be put into practice. The view of diagnosis described in the preceding pages is actually quite simple and can guide any busy clinician in his or her work.

In considering a diagnostic question, the practitioner considers three elements: the biomedical aspect of the problem, the psychosocial factors, and the relationship between the two.

THE BIOMEDICAL CORE

Physicians are always concerned with the physical aspects of their patients' problems. To do otherwise would break the patients' trust. Why else would patients go to doctors, except that they sense their expertise in such matters? The practitioners' skill is their sense of balance and appropriateness. They are always alert to the biomedical aspects of the patient's complaint. To "start" from some other place when the patient presents a physical complaint—i.e., to leap to the psychosocial aspects of each problem—would be a mistake. Not only would it be one-sided and dogmatic, but it would be a misrepresentation of the practitioner's role.

The physician's task is to *serve* his or her patients, on their terms, if possible. Thus, the clinician shows concern with the patient's somatic problems and respects them. Furthermore, science and technology have

91

made great advances in the past hundred years, which cannot be tossed aside, and which, in fact, have contributed to each practitioner's prestige and reputation. These advances must be well integrated into the contemporary clinician's approach. It would be foolish to claim that medical knowledge is an illusion or that medical skill does not exist or is mainly hurtful (as Illich does)—that makes each practicing physician a charlatan and con-man, and this is simply not the case. If physicians believe that they possess useful knowledge and skills, then they must preserve them and use them wisely.

The appreciation of the biomedical content of the patient's problem is the starting point for the clinician. It is the core of current medical practice, and the basis for the contract between physician and patient.

Having said this, it is clear that some biomedical problems are relatively easy to diagnose, while others are more difficult, and some appear to have no clear-cut answer at all. Simple diagnoses often lead to simple treatment. Complicated diagnoses may make management more difficult. But the diagnosis is always in a stage of evolution, and even complicated or obscure problems may become simple at some point in time, while a "simple" problem often has a way of splitting into a thousand different pieces.

The student of medicine needs to feel more at ease with uncertainty and change, for this is the nature of medical practice, illness, and people's lives. At any given point, a working diagnosis can be made and pursued, and it can always be amended if it has not been presented as the "last word" from the beginning.

Often, however, the "working diagnosis" is not satisfactory if it sticks to only biomedical problems, to "disease." Perhaps it seems to miss the point of the patient's having come. Perhaps it leads to severe problems of compliance and change. At times like these, both patient and practitioner must broaden or deepen the diagnosis by including other considerations in it, considerations which will usually come from an interactional or psychosocial perspective.

THE PSYCHOSOCIAL ENVELOPE

Psychosocial factors can be conceived as forming rings which envelop the biomedical core (Figure 11), thus helping the physician understand the illness better. This level of understanding comprehends many other factors which affect the course of illness, its management, its exacerbation or relapse. The broader level may even redefine the problem, as when an anxiety state is reformulated in terms of the family dynamics, or when the appearance of an ulcer right after the loss of a wanted job is understood as a reactive illness.

The psychosocial dimensions usually focus on the *context* of the problem and on the *interaction* occurring around it. Description deepens understanding of process. Grasping the systemic pattern may help a clinician touch upon the different meanings the illness carries in a particular family.

In terms of the hierarchy of systems, while the biomedical approach is concerned mainly with the molecular, cellular, humoral, organ, or organ system level, the psychosocial approach is concerned mainly with social units composed of one or more people, and thus with interactional patterns and dynamics.

THE RELATIONSHIP BETWEEN THE TWO

In its simplest sense, psychosomatic medicine is concerned with the relationship between physical illness and its psychosocial surround. This is what concerns us, too, as we view illness from a contextual or systemic perspective. The relationship between family (and other contextual)

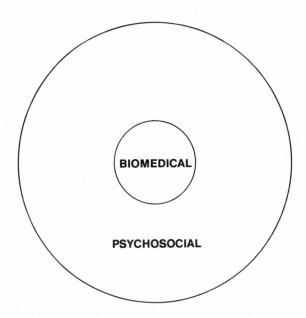

Figure 11. Diagnosis: Biomedical core, psychosocial envelope.

On Diagnosis

stresses and the patterns of illness that emerge is at the heart of both diagnosis and treatment.

Indeed, we are now finding that more and more areas of overlap exist, as in current stress research (Ader, 1982). Further areas of overlap will be found as research proceeds. Thus, it is critically important for clinicians to continue pursuing the broader perspectives, seeking out inter-relationships between levels of systems—environment, family, workplace, early experience, memories, family patterns, fears, etc.

After all, our world is a world of many systems, like a set of Chinese boxes, one inside the other, each of which can affect our well-being at any time. Physicians can choose to define their work as narrowly as possible, finding a measure of fulfillment at doing a modest job well, and renouncing any broader ambition or responsibility. Or they can choose the broader perspective, in the interests of being better prepared to help figure out and treat their patients' problems. The former is the path to more and more specialization. The latter is the road to expanded primary care.

Now, as before, the clinician's task is to preserve an open mind about the patients who come for help, and to explore, with astuteness and curiosity, both the process in which he or she is involved and that vibrant web of sensation and feeling in which all of us define the meanings of our life.

Part II

Diagnosis as a Contract:
Illustrative Problems

CHAPTER 9

The Diagnosis as a Social Contract

Arrived at, in fact *created* through a social process, diagnosis can be seen as a contract between different parties. It is an agreement which highlights salient symptoms, names the disease process which has caused them, and outlines how to treat the patient. The diagnosis characterizes the patient's problem and places it in context, thus giving it meaning. It paves the way to treatment, and helps clarify the problem for others in the patient's family and social world. It can create or deny the social role of patient for the one who is suffering. The diagnosis expresses the physician's understanding of "the illness" and its treatment, and structures medical care, facilitating payment, organizing treatment, and assigning social roles to patient, family, and treating health personnel.

The diagnosis rapidly becomes a shared opinion. Usually, it is shared between the patient and the physician, but it often happens that other people are involved in agreements over diagnosis. Without such agreement, difficulties would surely emerge. For example, it would be difficult for a patient to continue with a physician if the groundwork for their relationship—some form of agreement about the meaning of the patient's suffering—has not been established. Similarly, in the absence of an agreement over diagnosis, effective treatment can hardly take place. The diagnostic contract is essential for therapeusis.

Different people can be involved in this process. The patient and physician usually form the core of any diagnostic contract, but the patient's family, employer, friends, and the rest of his or her social network can all establish contracts around a diagnosis, as can other members of the medical system—e.g., nurses, physician assistants. In so doing, these participants will also inevitably affect the data on which the diagnosis is based: the patient's complaints and subjective response to treatment. In addition, different diagnoses, albeit presumably based on the same "facts" around the same problem, may exist between different people at any given time.

Example 15

Clara A, a 78-year-old woman, was admitted from the emergency room with a diagnosis of "transient ischemic attacks." She had developed slurred speech and right-sided weakness. The emergency room doctor felt she should be immediately anticoagulated. The family physician did not. He felt the patient might have had a "stroke"—which might have been on the basis of a cerebral hemorrhage, in which case anticoagulation was contraindicated, or on the basis of a developing clot. He called for a neurological consultation. The specialist found that the patient was also complaining that she saw brightly flashing lights and visually moving objects. He postulated that something was affecting the patient's posterior circulation. A vascular surgeon was called in. Finding carotid bruits, he suspected that the patient was indeed having "transient ischemic attacks" as the emergency room physician had suspected, and he felt she was in danger of having a stroke unless her carotid arteries were surgically cleaned out.

The situation began to resemble the "blind men and the elephant." Each physician had a different view of the patient's problem. This was a diagnostic dilemma, with three or four different opinions in contention and treatment hanging in the balance. Patient and family were both extremely anxious and confused, which appeared to be an appropriate response to the medical disagreement.

CONFLICT

Disagreement stems from conflict: conflict in values, conflict in attitude, conflict in interpreting the patient's signs and symptoms. Following Freidson, we should understand that conflict is not only inherent in the physician-patient relationship, but it is often its dominant aspect.

In addition, it exists in all other human relationships, including those among colleagues and co-workers, and it holds even when the more humanistic physician (cf. Carmichael and Carmichael, 1982) desires a cooperative and mutual relationship with his or her patient. Conflict exists because people emerge from different contexts with competing, dissimilar needs and demands.

Conflict around diagnosis usually arises in three main areas: 1) questions of biomedical (or other) fact; 2) questions of evaluating the meaning of the illness; and 3) questions of treatment.

1) Questions of Biomedical Fact

Uncertainty confronts both physician and patient. How much testing is necessary to "uncover" the problem behind the symptoms, or to indicate that no such problem exists? How can test results, whether positive or negative, be interpreted? Different experts may understand the same findings differently; diagnosis is often a matter of opinion. The further along the spectrum of uncertainty, the greater the range for debate about the patient's problem.

Example 16

Gwen B, a 36-year-old woman, came to the emergency room with chest pain and was found to have an abnormal cardiogram. In spite of this, and mainly because of her youthful age and additional findings of tender ribs, the emergency room physician felt she had costochondritis, an inflammation of the ribs. Because the EKG was abnormal, however, he called in a cardiologist. The cardiologist felt the patient had a viral inflammation involving the heart's lining, and he put her in the ICU for observation. Miss B's family physician felt that, even in spite of her relatively young age, she might be experiencing severe crescendo angina pectoris. Such a diagnosis suggests a possibly impending heart attack.

Because of hospital policy, the patient was the cardiologist's responsibility in the ICU, and she was treated as having viral pericarditis. After two days, the cardiologist, feeling his diagnosis had been correct, released Miss B to the ward, but there she still complained of severe pains in her chest. The nursing staff commented on her "bizarre" personality and frequent requests for pain medications, implying she might be unstable or a drug addict.

Miss B's pains persisted. The family physician urged cardiac catheterization as a technique which could establish a cardiac diagnosis and possibly indicate a need for coronary artery surgery (if she was indeed in a pre-infarction state), to ward off a heart attack. The cardiologist recommended waiting.

This uncertainty around Miss B's diagnosis was resolved two days later when her pains suddenly stopped, and the EKG tracing showed the classic signs of an acute myocardial infarction.

2) Questions About the Meaning of the Illness

Once an illness has been established, the patient and the patient's family will come to many conclusions about its significance. They will decide what it was due to and what it connotes for the future. These assumptions may differ markedly from the physician's own understanding of the process. Ensuing rifts in understanding, creating uncertainty, unclarity, and difference, can become an open field for anxiety, blame, and guilt.

Conflict can arise directly or indirectly over the significance of the disease. Will the patient now have to limit his or her activities? Should someone else be guilty over having "caused" the problem? Should the patient blame himself for negligence in bringing about the illness? Is the illness hereditary? Will the patient now be susceptible to more and more frequent bouts of illness? What else does the diagnosis suggest for the patient and his or her family?

Example 17

Dan C was a 63-year-old man who had developed Alzheimer's disease, presenile dementia. His mental deterioration was rapid. He stammered and mumbled, forgot his words, and was grossly confused. Such behavior contrasted sharply with what he had been like only a few months earlier. His family could not believe the transformation. They constantly wondered if they had done something wrong to bring on the man's condition, or to aggravate it once it had begun. Had it been a nutritional problem? Would more vitamins have helped? Was it related to nerves and stress? Should they perhaps have been more considerate, encouraged him to work less hard, fewer hours? Was it because of family arguments, and in this sense were they all to blame for his condition?

Did Mr. C now need to be cared for? Did he need a nursing home; if not now, would he in the future; and if he would, how would they know when? Did they have to pamper him, try not to make him angry? Did they have to treat him like a baby? Could he be expected to do anything for himself, and if so, what? How far would they have to rearrange their own lives in order to accommodate his needs? Finally, they wondered if this kind of mental deterioration was something that all of them might now have to look forward to.

3) Questions of Treatment

Even when an illness appears relatively simple to diagnose, conflict can surface over issues of treatment and around the degree of incapacity, dislocation, and adjustment that the patient's family has to accept. For example, a patient may be diagnosed as having a diseased gall bladder after a single attack: Should the gall bladder be taken out surgically or remain in? A patient may be felt to have an irritable bowel syndrome: Should sedatives be prescribed or should treatment focus on dietary changes and counseling? A patient has had a stroke and claims she cannot walk: How much should her family encourage and "push" her to get on her feet again? Patients, physicians, consultants, and family members—all have different ideas about how any particular illness should be treated.

Conflict is a constant feature of life in medicine. Physicians may prefer to reframe it when it appears, as a problem of "difficult patients"—then anyone with a different idea than the physician is "difficult." This is because physicians often feel they need to preserve membership in their own guild at all costs. They prefer not to carry out disputes among themselves. Physicians often make errors of judgment. If disputes with their colleagues are carried out publicly, it can only lead to cycles of triumph and defeat. Today's victor will be tomorrow's fool, but all will look foolish in the public eye. Therefore, physicians have an interest in keeping their own relations as free from public conflict as possible and would rather perceive conflict as stemming from the destructive behavior of "difficult" patients.

Of course, the same process appears as a problem of "cold and insensitive doctors" to patients and their families. The problem is thus systemic. One's viewpoint follows one's interests. Conflict naturally stems from the clash of different perspectives and the different levels of understanding which accompany the work of coping with illness and physical distress.

This process can escalate in a runaway fashion. Uncertain or debatable diagnoses, or diagnoses which conceal moral and ethical opinions, can actually set physicians fighting with one another, organize family members against physicians, fragment a ward's nursing staff into two camps, set nurses against a treating physician, or embroil participants in litigation, recrimination, and difficult wranglings which involve, at their broadest extension, the welfare system, the schools, the courts; hospitals, the insurance companies, medical societies, universities, and legislative bodies.

Example 18

Becky D, an attractive, 24-year-old married woman, had injured her right arm and leg in an auto accident. She was suing the other driver. She was also suing a local emergency room for allegedly failing to treat her correctly on the night of the accident. Now in another hospital, she was seen by Dr. Z, an orthopedic surgeon. He advised her to drop her suit. Miffed, Miss D asked Dr. Z's partner, Dr. Y, for an independent opinion, and then requested daily visits from him as well. Dr. Z became furious. He and Dr. Y engaged in a shouting match in the nurses' station. Subsequently, they asked the family physician to resolve their dispute by transferring the patient to a tertiary care teaching hospital where she could be treated by another "neutral" orthopedic surgeon. This was done, much to the patient's anger and irritation. All physicians agreed that Miss D had been a *very* "difficult patient."

PLURALISTIC CONTEXT

The family practitioner's usual day involves contracting complicated, multiple, or coexisting diagnoses with a number of different people: the patient, concerned family members, employers, insurance companies, the state, various bureaucratic agencies, and so on. The context for diagnosis and treatment is thus broadly pluralistic. Many forces converge around the identified patient's designated medical problem(s).

This is another reason why treatment becomes impossible without at least a minimal contract. Who will pay for such care? Most reimbursement depends on a stated diagnosis. Some hospital payments (Medicare) are now being organized "prospectively," which means that the payment is fitted to the admitting diagnosis, not to the unique peculiarities of the patient's condition. Any therapeutic intervention can then become a focus for further dispute. When patient and physician are "not on the same wave length," furthermore, misunderstandings are sure to occur; and family members will enter the scene, angry and hurt, confused, accusatory, and pushing for an answer to their universal question, "Hey, doc. What's the story with—? What's going *on*?"

Much patient dissatisfaction with physicians is said to result from the physician's "lack of communication." The patient or family member claims that the physician has failed to explain what the problem "really" is, and what can be done about it. Or that the physician has given only general instructions about treatment, neglecting the specifics of what can be done. Or that he or she has failed to grasp some aspect of the sickness or its treatment, which is emotionally extremely disquieting to the patient and family.

Usually, however, the problem is not "lack of communication." Communication has been only too clear—but someone is not pleased with it. In other words, the physician has probably very well communicated her attitude about the problem, but the patient or someone close to the patient disagrees with what's been said. For example, the patient's family may want more information about the problem, but the physician may prefer to say little except that they should "trust" her judgment and skill, and that she will "let them know" if any problem comes up. They, of course, may feel that problems have already come up and are not being dealt with.

Another example might involve a patient's wanting a more particular answer to a question, which the physician brushes off. Or the patient may want the physician to ask how he feels about his symptoms, but the physician insists on pursuing a strictly biomedical workup, and avoids any inquiry into how the patient is experiencing it. This often emerges when a patient visits a consultant. The specialist feels her task is to "rule in" or "rule out" pathology in her field. She proceeds with the tests peculiar to her subspecialty—e.g., esophagogastroscopy, ERCP, etc.—and then renders a verdict. The patient, on the other hand, may feel like a tree in someone else's forest, "along for the ride" but never really noticed or spoken to. From this, resentment about the high-priced but taciturn and "cold" specialist is quick to follow.

This phenomenon, arising from the clash of different perceptions people bring with them into the medical arena, has been discussed under the "attributions" of illness (Mishler et al., 1981; Stoeckle and Barsky, 1980; Waitzkin and Stoeckle, 1976): different conceptions of what is wrong; what happened to make it so; what it signifies; and what ought to be done and by whom to make it right again.

Other factors can produce conflict, too. These include the differing values—ethical, moral, and personal—which each of us carries into the medical encounter, as well as the deeper meanings by which we judge the illness's significance and assess our own adequacy at coping with it. In addition, grounds for conflict include different class interests and cultural outlooks which mold our perspective, as well as differing "meaning patterns" which are shared by communities, religious and occupational groups, and even generational cohorts. Feelings about simple X-rays, for example, vary widely according to social class, age and education. Those who perceive nuclear energy, radiation of all forms, and technology as a threat to life are much less likely to go along with routine dental or chest X-rays. To the physician who takes the diagnostic value of such tests for granted and who is frequently not alarmed by such "minor" accumulations of radiation, such misgivings and worry on the part of the patient or his family may start the "problem patient" bell ringing.

We take it for granted that others see the world as we do, and think all sensible people believe what we believe. Yet many conflicts and dissatisfactions actually result from a clash of covert perspectives. A diagnostic contract which contains elliptical clauses, omissions, and misconceptions is very likely to offend or disappoint someone. A simple example of this would be a patient's expecting to be called with her lab results, while her physician intends to phone only if the results are abnormal. "I'll give you a call," the physician may say, understanding to herself: ". . . if there's a problem you should be concerned about." It is the simple, "natural" mistake which can make people worry "Why????" for hours.

Applying a systems approach to the single topic of diagnosis, we can begin to understand how complex even the simplest medical event really is. It involves acknowledging the differing perspectives which make up the pluralistic context. In taking this "long view," however, the student of diagnostic process must be both participant and observer. It does no good to observe from afar, pronouncing judgment on the inadequate actions of people involved in life's day-to-day decisions. A systems perspective should be a guide to practice. The diagnostician's activity is a relentless to-and-fro process: interaction with the patient and family; pulling back for reflection; re-immersion in order to ask questions and test hypotheses, hear the patient once again, and interact with the family; and once again pulling back to look at the process as a whole. Becoming fixed at either of these poles may lead to error. The physician lost in practical details fails to seek the overall picture and will not appreciate the shifting patterns. The too scholarly physician, aloof and detached, loses rapport with patients, and the "feel" of reality slips from her fingertips. Knowledge develops dialectically over time, in a continuing spiral (Mao Tse-tung, 1966).

We can now more closely examine the problems that arise when diagnosis is seen as a contract between members of different systems or between different members of the same system. The following discussion should again remind us how incomplete is any notion of diagnosis as a process entirely within the physician's own mind, and how difficult it is to pronounce what the patient is "really" suffering from. In the conflict of perspectives, "facts" are often exposed to be simply privileged, empowered opinion made socially legitimate.

CHAPTER 10

The Contract With Oneself:
The Special Example
of the Physician

The simplest kind of contract is the contract people make with themselves, like a promise to oneself or an inmost belief. Persons involved around an illness may each make such a contract with themselves, reflecting what they "really" think is going on. They may not share this belief with anyone else. When physicians make such a contract with themselves, they, too, are saying what they "really" feel is going on, a view which may not be recorded on any encounter form, but which represents their deepest sense of "what is wrong."

Many of the old-time GP's used to keep their records on small index cards. These were not "problem-oriented" charts. Instead, they were brief notes, weights and blood pressure readings, fragments of thought, billing notes. Most of what they understood was kept in their heads, and they tended not to share this information with anyone, neither patients nor colleagues. These were their private thoughts. For example, when someone asked the GP what the problem was, he might respond, "Well now, you let *me* worry about that." Or he might murmur something vague and nondescript like, "The idea, John, is that it's your circulation." Or, "You've got tired blood," or "It's a digestive disturbance."

In the quiet of his own mind, though, the GP formed a notion of the problem. Such notions are hard to get at today, but the contemporary physician can certainly recognize the feeling that whatever is written on the form, whatever is communicated in letters or reports, and whatever is conveyed in one way or another to the patient or to family members are somehow only approximations, bastardized versions of what he really understands "deep down" in his heart; what is communicated is just an abbreviation of the whole, written for the insurance company's benefit or to "give a handle on the illness" to someone who has asked for it.

After all, there is only so much room on any encounter form, only so many blanks in an insurance questionnaire, and only so much that any patient or family member can grasp. But the physician, who has all the lab data, X-ray reports, and his own examination—history and physical, both—to draw upon, feels he has a more complicated, more intricate understanding of what the problem is. As soon as he has to share this with someone, though, it becomes less complete: The whole can never be communicated. How, for example, does he convey those intangible sensations and feelings the patient arouses in him in the course of the presentation, evaluation, and treatment of this illness? How can he, trained in the medical sciences, but not in verbal skills, sum up or express what he feels?

The same feeling, the same conviction, holds for each person with a private view, physician or someone else. It holds for the patient, the patient's mother, the nurse on the ward where the patient is hospitalized, the secretary who knows the patient's family, and so on. This is a little acknowledged fact which lies at the heart of many later disputes.

The physician, like others, cannot fully express his inner conviction, and, as a consequence, may prefer to keep his feelings to himself. This would not concern us here but for one fact: Such feelings form much of the basis for his subsequent management of this patient and her illness. What the physician believes deep down may or may not jibe with what he tells the patient. It may or may not jibe with what he has written down on the insurance paper or in the letter to the patient's employer asking for another month out of work. It is something peculiar to himself, something private and relatively inaccessible, and something which determines his own behavior.

Because it is such a private thing, this kind of diagnostic impression cannot be much discussed. But its effects are important. It forms the unspoken substrate upon which many physicians' comments and acts depend. It is often inferred by the patient, guessed at in an attempt to figure out why the doctor did what he did; others may also make attempts to figure out what the physician "really" believes. Because of its secrecy, though, this diagnostic view can almost always also be misunderstood and guessed at erroneously.

The physician's diagnosis also reflects his own value system. If he views suffering as an inevitable part of life, expecting people to deal with it stoically, as he perhaps does, he will be less inclined to grant disabilities and place people on the welfare rolls. On the other hand, if he is more sympathetic to the struggles of his patients against the "adverse" forces of life, viewing himself as their protagonist, he may yield to the diagnosis of a disabling injury or process much more readily.

If the physician tends to view illness as a mainly physical problem, he will tend to underdiagnose the depression, anxiety, and fears that his patients live with and develop. On the other hand, if he tends to see psychosocial forces everywhere, he may gloss over physical problems while eagerly encouraging his patients to speak about their conflicts and feelings. In this and other ways, the physician's attitude may conflict with that of his or her patient.

When the physician's values jibe with those of his patient, however, there will usually be more harmony between the two of them, a higher degree of both physician and patient satisfaction (Roger Bibace, personal communication, 1983). In addition, they will both find it easier to discuss those values which underlie their decisions. When the physician's values differ from the patient's, even though each may notice this, it is less likely to be openly discussed, and remains a matter of "personal opinion."

Are there reasons today for physicians to maintain a private diagnostic view today? I think there are. The main reason stems from their often isolated and lonely conditions of work: The solo practitioner, still the most common practitioner in the U.S. today, cannot share his impressions with anyone. He cannot gossip to his staff about patients. He cannot tell his spouse anecdotes from work without breaking his patients' confidentiality. And, since he feels other physicians have a tendency to judge him by the stories he tells, he usually feels odd simply sharing an observation or perspective with his colleagues.

Thrust onto a pedestal both by his own training and by the deferential behavior of those around him, he tends to regard his most secret opinions as incontestably true. Through this both grandiose and defensive world outlook, one can discern the paranoia-engendering effects of social isolation, of not having to share a viewpoint with others. Nevertheless, the physician, much like the rest of us, clings to what is most hidden in his own heart; it would, further, be wrong to dismiss the acumen which has also contributed to his personal judgments about his patients' suffering. Because this entity, however, can only be guessed at—it becomes an interpersonal communication as soon as we ask about it—we shall leave it, merely mentioned and described, lurking in the background, as are everyone else's inner thoughts, as we pursue the more observable forms of social contracts around diagnosis.

CHAPTER 11

The Contract Between Patient and Physician

As we have seen, the patient presents a diversity of symptoms to the physician. Considering them, the physician selects a diagnosis to pursue. It may or may not be the one that most concerns the patient. It may be the one the physician feels most comfortable about pursuing, or the one he feels most worried about, because of its prognosis. In any case, this response lays the basis for the subsequent patient-physician contract. It also contains the seeds of their future conflict.

Because of the physician's professional role, status, and reputation, the patient usually has to go along with his judgment. For example, if the physician diagnoses the problem as an emergency and recommends urgent treatment, the patient can do little except comply or change physicians. Negotiating is possible only when the situation is not serious, or when alternative approaches bear equivalent risks or side-effects and offer similar benefits:

Example 19

Hal D had gone through surgery for stones in his left ureter and kidney. A rubber tube had been placed from his kidney area to an incision in his flank, so any excessive fluid would not accumulate. But the tract created by this drain continued to leak urine-like fluid, even after it was supposed to have healed, and weeks after the patient had been discharged from the hospital. The drainage persisted and became worse, taking on a cloudy, purulent appearance. Mr. D had to be rehospitalized and was seen by another urologist. His fever was 102°, and he was having shaking chills. The second urologist diagnosed impending sepsis (infection in the bloodstream), a very dangerous problem. He therefore recommended immediate surgery to explore the area of the operation, feeling that the ureter was blocked off, which forced the urine out the sinus tract.

But Mr. D did not want an operation. He wanted to wait. He was not at all sure this new doctor was right, and he wanted to wait until the doctor who performed the operation returned from vacation. The second urologist, however, would not hear of this: "In my opinion, this is a very dangerous matter," he said. "You could go into shock at any time. You could run a temperature of 105°. You could die. If you refuse to have the operation, I cannot be responsible for your care, and you will have to speak to whoever else is covering for Dr. J [who performed the original surgery]."

After heated discussion with his wife, Mr. D agreed to the operation. He said it was foolish to argue over the diagnosis or to wait three days for a "second opinion." After all, according to the second urologist, who was now treating him and who had to be listened to, he was in serious condition and could not afford to wait.

The contract between patient and physician often reflects this power difference. Earlier, we saw how physician-patient relationships differ according to how active and authoritarian the physician chooses to be, how much control and voice the patient expects to have, and how each deals with the other's expectations of his own and the other's behavior. The balance of control between the two shapes their contract.

Some patients offer: "Doc, do whatever you think is right. I'll do whatever you say." Their contract involves giving up all responsibility and simply following the physician's directions. In exchange, the doctor agrees to assume control, to "take charge" and do his best.

Other patients will not feel comfortable without an active part in the contract. They need to help negotiate their diagnosis and subsequent treatment plan.

Some patients, like the old-time GP mentioned earlier, will form their own diagnosis, their own understanding of what has gone wrong and why, and keep it to themselves. Their secret understanding may carry profound meaning, and may actually be one of their main ways of dealing with the illness.

Other conflicts can develop over what constitutes adequate preventive medical measures, when the treatment of a given illness might have gone too far, and when the picture of an illness is complete. The patient's agenda differs from the physician's, but the two of them often wish to avoid recognizing this, neither wishing to make the conflict explicit. In order to work together and maintain the relationship, however, they must agree on some aspect of treatment.

THE NECESSITY FOR MAKING THE CONTRACT

The contract between doctor and patient requires agreeing on something. For example, the two may agree to deal with a particular set of symptoms. They may agree on a diagnosis. They may agree on a course of treatment, whatever the diagnosis. They may agree that there is no clear-cut diagnosis, and that even the problems are unclear, but that they will continue to meet and discuss how the patient feels, simply maintaining access to one another.

Unless there is some kind of agreement, however, each of them is dancing in his own world, with his own idea of what is wrong and what it signifies. Their activity is not coordinated. Further, without a mutual contract each is likely to misunderstand the other's intent and thoughts, and their relationship is jeopardized. The failure to establish an overt contract can lead to covert conflict.

For example, in a case referred to earlier, a patient suffering from a benign eye condition is incidentally found to have a cancer of the lung. The physician is eager, and feels professionally bound, to investigate this positive finding. Perhaps he can make the diagnosis early enough to save the patient's life. But, to his dismay, the patient not only refuses this invitation for further workup, referral, and biopsy, but becomes angry to the point of being violent, bellicose, and refusing any further contact with the physician.

The patient says, "The only thing bothering me is my blurred vision, which I want fixed. I don't have any pain in my chest. I don't have any trouble breathing. Okay, so I have this cough, which is the same cough I've had for the last seven years. If I start to feel badly, I'll come in and see you. But right now, I don't want to."

The physician sends the patient a letter, saying how serious his condition is. He phones the patient's wife, trying to enlist her aid. He knows the patient is "denying" the problem, probably out of deep-seated fear of acknowledging the cancer. But what can he do? His hands are tied.

The contract is impossible if the patient and physician cannot agree, or if they cannot agree on how to handle their disagreement. For example, both may agree that the patient is very likely suffering from bursitis of the shoulder. Or, supposing that they disagree, they can still agree that the patient will try a certain medicine for a week, obtain X-rays, and pursue further consultation if the pain does not respond in ten days.

They may disagree on a diagnosis, but agree on treatment. They may disagree on both the diagnosis and the treatment, but agree on the severity of the illness's meaning and significance to the patient. Thus, there are many potential levels at which they can establish a working link. Lacking any such level, they may agree that they will disagree for a time being, and "take turns" in guiding the treatment and workup. The physician may order tests because the patient's wife earnestly wishes him to order them; or the patient may grudgingly accept a course of treatment because the physician earnestly feels it merits at least a chance. My simple point is that they have to agree on *something*.

Thus they can agree; agree to disagree; agree by ceding; pretend to agree; agree there are no grounds for agreeing; and even imagine that they are agreeing, when in fact each believes something quite different. It doesn't matter—each of these alternatives provides at least a basis for the contract, a basis for further treatment.

OTHER OBSTACLES TO THE CONTRACT

Many obstacles may prevent the physician and patient from coming to an agreement:

1) They may disagree on the *hierarchy of complaints*: The patient may feel that his chest pain is his most serious problem, while the physician may be worried more about a certain blood finding, or feel that the chest pain only signals the degree of emotional tension the patient is experiencing, which is the "real" problem.
2) Patient and physician may have different *expectations* of how they both should proceed. The patient may want to talk about his or her problems and understand them better. But the physician, pressed for time, may want only to prescribe medicines and have the patient return later. Each may see both his and the other's role differently, and thus not go along with the other's expectations. Further, if the patient disagrees with the physician's view and expects something different, he may be perceived as a "bad" patient.
3) This is closely connected to the problem that patient and physician may have different *agendas*. For example, the patient may want the

physician to give him pain-killers and a welfare form, but the physician may want to diagnose whether the patient has "real" back pain
or not.

4) The patient and physician may understand the same terms and illness
differently: Their *attributions* may be at odds with one another. If the
physician diagnoses an ulcer, the patient who imagines that an ulcer
means imminent death from vomiting blood will fight the diagnosis
and deny it.

5) Different attributions can stem from *cultural and class differences*. These
obstacles interfere with the establishment of a contract because the
physician and patient are literally speaking different languages, which
connote different things to one another.

6) Yet another obstacle comes up when the physician questions the
validity of the patient's complaints: *skepticism and disbelief*. Feeling that
the physician does not believe what he says, the patient is less inclined
to accept what the physician has to say.

7) Finally, the fact of many complaints, many illnesses, can overwhelm
both the patient and physician. The focus shifts and skips so much
that the two have difficulty getting on the same wave length. The
patient complains of headache; the physician inquires; the patient
then begins talking about dyspepsia; the physician, remembering the
last meeting they had, inquires about chest pains; the patient mini-
mizes that complaint, but talks instead of "wicked" headaches; the
physician starts to scribble a prescription for headaches; the patient
interrupts by racing for the scale and complaining that he can't possibly lose weight, and how can that be, since he is always nauseated
and never can eat a bite; and so on.

Consider, for instance, the case of the woman quoted in Section I:
"Oy, doctor, you got a sick woman on your hands. My heart pounds.
My head aches. I got a burnin' in my stomach . . ." (p. 33). The physician
might conceivably make a contract with the patient for each particular
complaint. For example, the patient might be sent to a number of specialists, one for the heart, one for the joints, one for the stomach, one
for the headache, one for the depression. Perhaps she will agree to talk
about the whole gestalt at some later time, but for the present she is not
interested in that. She is interested in each particular organ system which
she feels is disintegrating, and she wants to know "why" this is so, and
what can be done about it.

Let us cite again what Claude Bernard (1957) said about asking "why":

The nature of our mind leads us to seek the essence or the *why* of things. Thus we aim beyond the goal that is given us to reach; for experience soon teaches us that we cannot get beyond the *how*, i.e., beyond the immediate cause or the necessary conditions of phenomena. . . . (p. 80)

Physiologists and physicians must therefore always consider organisms as a whole and in detail at one and the same time, without ever losing sight of the peculiar conditions of all the special phenomena whose resultant is the individual. (p. 91)

This is an example of how concern with first-order change (cf. the later discussion on p. 000) only perpetuates the problem, while concern with second-order change—how to approach the problem and conceptualize it—offers the only hope for altering the problem. In this case, approaching the patient's entire set of problems as a pattern of complaining would lead to the main issue, how the woman expresses depression and worry in many bodily ways. One might then deal with her use of the physician, her feelings, and so on, and *bypass* the need for dealing with each particular distressing symptom.

CONFLICT AROUND THE MIND/BODY DICHOTOMY

One type of conflict especially difficult to overcome involves arguments over the mind/body dichotomy. When the physician senses that part of the problem is "emotional," but the patient insists that the entire problem is "physical," the two will be in for a difficult time, especially if the physician is unable to translate his concern and perception into "body language."

The patient with many somatic symptoms which appear to be related to anxiety, but who denies being anxious, is a classic "difficult patient." Even if she eventually admits that she is anxious, she will probably say this is only "because of" her wretched physical condition, her palpitations, tight stomach, headache, and so on, all of which *must* be due to some physical condition. Sometimes, such patients can understand the connection of their physical symptoms to their level of anxiety, but often they simply cannot. A few examples will clarify how this arises in practice:

Example 20

Sally F had developed pains throughout her body. In addition, she was dizzy, and complained of palpitations, numb fingers, tingling cheeks, gasping for air, and so on. She also had pains over her heart, diarrhea, stomachaches, neck pains, and cramps. The physician "read" these as signs of anxiety and hyperventilation syndrome.

"Why is my back stiff? Why does my heart beat so fast? Do I have heart disease? Why am I dizzy? Is it a tumor in my head? Do I have an aneurysm? God, I hope I'm not going to die. Am I going to die? Why do my fingers get so cold and numb? Why?" she would say.

Groping, the physician tried: "All these feelings come on because you're upset. They're bodily signs of tension, of being worried. It's not your heart, Sally, it's . . ."

"It's not in my head," she insisted.

"But I didn't say it was in your head. I know it's not in your head. It's because you're so upset. Because you're under so much tension because of the job, your mother, the things you think about all the time. . . . Your muscles get tense when you feel that way, and . . ."

"So you're saying it's in my head. But it isn't. There's something wrong there. I'm not under any stress or tension or whatever you call it. I mean, I may be, but I'm tense because I'm sick. You'd be, too. My marriage is fine. My job is hectic, but I can handle it."

And then the inevitable argument: "You think you're upset because of all the pain. I understand that. But I think," the doctor says, "that you're having all these pains because you're upset."

"I understand, too. You think it's in my head. I know it's in my body."

"The body reacts to stress and tension . . ."

"That's not what's going on. If you want to know what's going on, do something. Take an EKG. Check my pulse. Give me an upper GI series. I don't know. Maybe I should see a neurologist. . . ."

And on it goes. Arguing over "which came first," the two fail to examine their own interchange at the next higher level. They do not see that they are arguing over two parts of the same process, and they do not discuss their arguing as a symptom in itself. Their relationship becomes a battle for control, a battle of prestige and self-esteem. The patient is boxed-in, unable to give in without losing her integrity. Contesting the diagnosis, the two are unable to work together.

Yet, to pursue countless tests, as Mrs. F demands, will also lead nowhere. It will cost thousands of dollars, inflict possible pain and suffering, and delay the recognition that the problem is indeed a mind/body problem, whose solution requires an integrative approach. If such a patient finds a frustrated physician who pursues the biomedical model, she may make a contract to spend thousands of dollars in a search for "real" physical illness, a search which may bring Mrs. F to within an inch of her life in such procedures as cardiac catheterization. Or, more likely, she will have surgery on some internal organs, in the hope that their malfunction is causing her pain.

She may accumulate a wide variety of physical diagnoses, but will probably still refuse to deal with the emotional aspect of her symptoms, which the first physician was correct in sensing. Is there a way the physician can more expertly "talk her language" without getting into a fight? Some people, especially some therapists used to working with people with somatic pains, feel there may be; but, at present, most physician-practitioners have little sense of it, and feel constantly frustrated at patients like Mrs. F, who either receive unnecessary treatments or break off and see another physician.

In retrospect, it is rarely wise to argue with a patient about a diagnosis. The argument turns into a battle for control, which is not helpful to either party.

Sometimes the difference between physician and patient will be so severe, the gap cannot be bridged without destroying the relationship. Then, the physician may have to choose between "truth and honesty" or "managing the patient and the illness" as best he can.

Example 21

Peg G was a 68-year-old widowed woman who insisted on vitamin B-12 injections and estrogen shots. She was convinced that these kept her healthy. In addition, she insisted on coming to the physician every week for these shots. If the physician would not give them to her, she said she would go elsewhere. In the brief weekly visits, she would sigh and talk about the dismal conditions of her life; but, when the subject of depression was raised *per se*, she would vigorously insist, "I'm not depressed. Oh, no. That's not me."

The physician was in a dilemma. To pursue the view that the patient was "depressed" would have led to further argument, explanation, and struggle for agreement. The patient might have left the practice and gone "down the street" to another physician who would have obliged her requests. To accede to her wishes meant the physician's having to stifle what he knew and give placebo injections, but with the aim of maintaining access to the patient, so he could be of use to her in times of emotional difficulty as well as in times of (real) physical illness. Such a dilemma often exists in the office of the family physician.

Example 22

Jackie H, a 27-year-old separated mother of two, consulted a new physician for severe back pain. She said she had sprained her back so badly that she could no longer go about her activities. She was given Valium and Percodan for several days, as well as muscle relaxants and non-steroidal anti-inflammatory drugs, but her disability persisted. She claimed she could not go to and from the hospital every day for physical therapy, and so she was hospitalized for further evaluation and treatment.

In the hospital, she demanded to be "knocked out." She asked again for Percodan and Valium, but these were not given to her. She was instead given physical therapy, muscle relaxants, analgesia, injections, and bedrest. After ten days, she was "no better." The nurses noted that she was constantly somnolent. Social service noted that she was separated, and that her angry husband continually berated the nursing staff for not caring enough for her. She was querulous and bitter, insistent on getting her pain medication, and quick to deny any reliance on it. After normal X-rays of the spine, normal EMG's, and normal blood work, the physician wondered at her total lack of improvement. She demanded Percodan and Valium again. The social worker learned that she had a six-year history of Valium and Percodan abuse, and a Valium overdose ten years ago when she was still a teenager.

Because of this lack of improvement and her considerable history of abuse, unhappy marriage, and domestic problems, psychotherapy was suggested. She reacted to it as if it was an insult, and angrily rejected the idea. "You'd be angry and unhappy, too, if you were me," she said. "But that's got nothing to do with my back pain. What's the matter with you? Don't you know what's wrong? You're the doctor, aren't you? If you are, then why can't you make me better? What do I have to do, live like this forever? I want you to do something to help me. You're my doctor. I don't need no headshrinker." She again asked to be "knocked out." Her husband began making angry phone calls to the physician, demanding to know why she was not better.

Finally, pain medications were tapered and stopped (she was half unconscious from them), and she was asked to rely on physical therapy. An angry scene ensued where she said, "Then I may as well go home." She cried that people were treating her like an addict; she was simply in pain and "nobody was doing anything to help" her.

She had repeatedly created the scenario of her being a helpless sufferer, being refused medication and treatment by a cruel medical world. Yet her response to treatment did not jibe with her claimed diagnosis. Her behavior in the hospital struck physicians and nurses alike as inappropriate. She was observed climbing over the side rails and walking with no limp at all, when she thought no one was watching. All medical personnel agreed that she was suffering from severe emotional problems, which she was refusing to face. She was therefore discharged.

Immediately after leaving the hospital, she came to the physician's office demanding Percodan, and threatening a malpractice suit if she did not receive it.

Here, the problem was breaking through the use of narcotics and sedatives as a soporific from an unhappy life. The basis for the patient-physician relationship could not be established. The patient wanted only drugs, and refused any other "offer." The physician could not in good conscience prescribe narcotics as "treatment" for this troubled woman. The diagnostic contract shattered, and so did the relationship.

No problem so taxes both the physician and the patient as the patient, like Jackie H, with a somatic disorder felt to be "caused by" or linked to emotional stress and worry. So strong is our conceptualization of physical illness as separate from emotional stress—in spite of all the conventional wisdom to the contrary—and so deep is the somaticizing patient's usual refusal to look at any but the physical aspects of her distress, that unravelling and reintegrating the problem become very hard.

The problem has been helped by the recent acknowledgment of somatoform disorders in DSM-III. One particular disorder is Briquet's syndrome. Variously diagnosed earlier as hysterical hypochondriasis, severe neurasthenia with borderline features, somatic obsessional disorder, and so on, this category of problem patient is well-known to all practitioners. Whatever contract can be made must occur at a meta-level—dealing not with the symptoms but with the treating relationship itself.

Example 23

Paula I was 25. She had seen another physician for many years, but he was entering semi-retirement and she was now being handed over to his new associate. She lived with her father, a hard-driving union official, and a younger sister, her mother having died when she was 17. Over the past three-year period she had displayed a remarkable variety of symptoms: The left half of her body went completely numb. She had chronic pains in her left knee, which had been arthroscoped in the past, and operated on for torn cartilage, and which had "never stopped killing" her. She complained of severe back pain, ever since an auto accident ten years earlier, which had been tentatively diagnosed as a ruptured disc, but for which there had been little evidence in repeated follow-up examinations. She also complained of persistent and irregular vaginal bleeding, and "black discharge." Her most persistent complaint was exquisite pain and swelling in her left thigh, which had been repeatedly diagnosed as "phlebitis" and for which she had taken blood-thinners from time to time. Reviewing her venous studies for the past six years, however, the new physician could find no positive tests. In addition, she was overweight and "could not lose a pound," even though she ate "no more than 800 calories a day." She also experienced frequent nausea, headaches, urinary infections, drowsiness, and general episodes of "just feeling completely lousy."

She denied any emotional problems and refused to talk to a counselor. She demanded physical examination of all her complaints. When confronted with other physicians' advice that she should have a psychiatric consultation, she grew morose, and said she didn't like those doctors and never wanted to see them again.

Her father stood staunchly behind her in denying the need for psychiatric treatment. "What are you saying? That she's nuts?" he demanded. "Well, if she's nuts, then I'm nuts, too."

The older physician had given Miss I vitamin injections, hormones, progesterone, steroids, diuretics, and anticoagulants. He had sent her to a number of specialists, responding quickly to each new complaint. In addition, whenever she had complained of back pain or "phlebitis," he had hospitalized her. In effect, however, he had allied himself with the patient's resistance to change: Seeking change in terms of her physical complaints, he had tried to make her feel better physically, but this had only perpetuated the situation. He had not tried to change the way she complained, had not attempted to *restructure* her illness. This was not a mistake on his part: He had not understood the problem in a systemic way, but continued to function as a concerned physician, thus unknowingly placing himself in a "reactive" position. Although it seemed that he, the physician, had the knowledge and power, he was actually being manipulated by Miss I. In fact, his role as the sympathetic, kindly family doctor kept the problem going. Following this role, he had no choice but to react "medically" when she came in with her usual complaints.

The course became complex over the next few months. Miss I was found to have a hypogonadotrophic hypogonadism, a hormonal insufficiency which explained her menstrual irregularities and her constant vaginal bleeding. She was sent to a major tertiary care center where, for a time, she was evaluated for a tumor of the pituitary gland, which, it turned out, she did not have. The menstrual difficulties, persistent complaints, and failure to respond to any course of hormonal medication, however, led her to undergo a hysterectomy before the age of 30, a decision which was most likely correct.

Her obesity became so grave a problem that she finally underwent gastric stapling for it, although she rejected concomitant counseling. She then complained that the surgeons had "botched" the job, and came to the office with recurrent nausea and vomiting, abdominal pains ("Do you think it's adhesions?"), and diarrhea. She received so many X-rays that the radiologist refused to perform any more on her.

Repeatedly, she sought orthopedic and vascular consultation on her own. She began to appear at the emergency rooms of local hospitals with vague stories—seizures, numbness, total body weakness. She was often admitted to hospitals by physicians who did not know her. Her case became incredibly difficult to "contain." It then became suspect that she was abusing pain medications and sedatives, and that some of her "seizures" might actually have been caused by withdrawal from these medications.

She had a talent for continually dragging someone else into the picture. If the new physician took a strong line with her, she would phone the previous physician. Or she would have her father gruffly phone, scolding the new doctor for not believing her. Or she would get a friend of the family to call, swearing that she was basically a "good kid." Or she would take herself, on her own, to see another consultant who would then institute a whole set of physical diagnostic tests, often without phoning the family doctor. Thus, she constantly managed to control her case. Confronted with such behavior, she would berate herself, apologize profusely, and beg the new doctor to continue to see her, as he was the "only" doctor who understood her, etc., etc. The new physician was slowly sliding into the same bind as his predecessor.

In spite of everything, she continued her weekly visits, complaining of her usual problems, and accepting vitamins. When the new doctor said that emotional problems were at the core of her distress, she would answer, "I know. It's all because my mother died. I wasn't ready. I loved her and I hated her, and that's that. So what else is new?"

The physician stopped pushing her to change and stopped responding to her chronic complaints. He tried instead only to observe that her youth was passing and that she must be feeling miserable about it. She responded by talking about her boyfriend, a job she was working "under the table," and her swimming pool at home. In spite of this, however, whenever life took a rough turn for her, she would present pale and sweaty, complaining of having eaten nothing for days, having lost 15 pounds, and begging for admission to the hospital.

It was clear that she deeply mourned her mother. She had even formed an attachment to one of the older patients in the practice whom she called "mother" and sent Mother's Day cards to. She was also obviously overinvolved with her father, whose task in life for the past ten years seemed to have been caring for his two daughters.

His valiant efforts finally collapsed, by the way, and he experienced both a stroke and a severe heart attack within a four-week period.

Miss I's problems continued. In a six-month period, she was hospitalized a number of times. On one occasion she required laparotomy, and was found to have a mass of adhesions. On another occasion, she had blood in her stool and was felt to be in the early stages of ulcerative colitis. On multiple occasions, she complained of flank pains and was found to have blood in her urine. Her course continues the same way to this day, with alternating episodes of "real" and unclear physical symptomatology.

This vignette shows how pursuing the medical diagnosis may only compound some problems, how pushing psychotherapy as an entirely separate endeavor is doomed to rejection, and how the physician is often so intimately involved himself in the whole system of physical complaints, response, and treatment, that he is little help in changing it. That is, he is so caught up that all his efforts at changing the problem involve "first-order changes." These only perpetuate the problem, and in fact come to *constitute* the problem. The only hope is to change the way the problem is perceived, to effect "second-order change."

The issue of control is critical here. So is the role of the other medical-care providers, whose insistence on a physical diagnosis presents the patient with a ready "out" whenever she needs it. The only tack that appeared to work here was continuing to see the patient while ignoring all her physical symptoms, and inquiring instead into her activities and relationships.

WHEN THE PATIENT IS "PSYCHOTIC"

The problem is compounded when the physician feels the patient is not mentally competent. Here, a "mutual" or collateral relationship appears impossible, because the physician has a secret which he cannot share with the patient.

Example 24

Yvette J, a 75-year-old woman, was convinced her family was trying to poison her. Living alone, she was in constant dread that someone would kill her, because she "knew" that her sister had poisoned her mother 11 years earlier.

She would appear in the physician's office with a bottle of urine, pleading, "Please. I want you to analyze this. You're the only one I can trust. They've put something in my food. It doesn't taste right. My urine is dark. I want you to find out what they put in my food."

The physician could only commiserate with her anxiety and fear. She refused to take tranquilizers. She refused any idea of counseling ("What I really need is a detective. But I can't call one up myself, you see, because they've tapped the telephone lines. . . ."). It appeared, though, that she gained something from coming in every month or two, weeping for a few minutes about how frightened she was to be the target of so much scheming. The physician continued to see her for her "blood pressure" in order simply to maintain access to her, which proved helpful when the patient contracted pneumonia and had to be hospitalized.

PROBLEMS WITH UNCERTAINTY

Many problems in primary-care practice are unclear. Their diagnosis may require lengthy observation, treatment, and testing. This task requires patient and physician to agree on how to approach the question. Even so, areas of uncertainty may remain and must be dealt with. Uncertainty over diagnosis can easily lead to a rift over how to proceed with treatment. Conflicting ideas about the "real" problem often cannot be objectively resolved and end up as different opinions about the diagnosis.

Example 25

Peter K complained of pains in his left shoulder. His job involved heavy manual work, and a tentative diagnosis of bursitis was made. His pains did not respond to a two-week course of the usual medications prescribed for this ailment. The physician then proposed a further workup, looking into other, non-orthopedic causes of Mr.

K's distress. He felt he might have heart trouble, gall bladder disease, or even troubles involving nervous tension or muscle spasm. "I'm not sure," he said. "Why don't we really look into this?"

But the patient did not agree. "No," he said. "How about giving me an injection in the shoulder, right where it hurts. Dr. B gave me one five years ago, and it seemed to help."

"I could do that," the physician mused. "But, to tell you the truth, Pete, I'd rather go for the full workup now."

"Well, if you don't want to give me the shot," the patient replied, "I'll go over to Dr. Fergusson. I know he's good with the needle."

Such dilemmas often arise in medical treatment. Decisions on surgery, decisions on the most appropriate treatment, decisions on further tests and procedures—CT scans, barium enemas, venograms, chemotherapy, arteriograms, biopsies, etc.—arise and create tension and strain. Usually, these dilemmas are linked to the same differences in perspective, level of understanding, and attributions of meaning (e.g., to a particular diagnostic test) that generate conflicts over diagnosis.

GETTING OUT OF BINDS: TWO KINDS OF CHANGE

Often, as we have seen, the physician finds himself "locked in" by what the patient believes. His repeated attempts to understand or to ameliorate the problem become part of the problem itself.

A systemic approach deals with this by distinguishing between "first-order" and "second-order" change. Watzlawick et al. have described this distinction as follows:

> . . . there are two different types of change: one that occurs within a given system which itself remains unchanged, and one whose occurrence changes the system itself. To exemplify this distinction in more behavioral terms: a person having a nightmare can do many things *in* his dream—run, hide, fight, scream, jump off a cliff, etc.—but no change from any one of these behaviors to another would ever terminate the nightmare. *We shall henceforth refer to this kind of change as first-order change.* The one way *out of* a dream involves a change from dreaming to waking. Waking, obviously, is no longer a part of the dream, but a change to an altogether different state. *This kind of change will from now on be referred to as second-order change.* (1967, pp. 10-11)

How does this concept help? When the physician and the patient are locked into a wrangle over diagnosis, the result is stagnation. The two are fighting for control. Attempts to change this pattern by "doing more of the same" will obviously not help. This is a "first-order change" approach: another set of blood tests, a CT scan, a barium enema with sigmoidoscopy, a new prescription for the complaints.

First-order change is called for when the problem appears correctly perceived and the physician and patient are simply trying to "hone in" on it more precisely. But when there is no pattern, and the struggle is proving hopeless, second-order change is called for. This amounts to commenting on the process itself, and holding it up for change. The physician might say: "We seem locked into ordering test after test, yet I wonder if these results will really help us figure out the problem." Or, "We've tried a whole series of different medications for this. Perhaps we should try taking you off *all* these medicines, see how you feel, and tackle the problem again."

An example of the solution becoming part of the problem is when the patient complains bitterly that the physician "is not doing anything" for him, which prompts the physician to order more tests, prescribe more drugs, and so on. Another example is the patient's rejecting the physician's request for psychiatric consultation, but demanding consultation with orthopedists, cardiologists, and so on.

Here are some examples of second-order change in the doctor-patient-family matrix:

1) Calling attention to the pattern of utilization of medical care: visits which seem unnecessary, repetitive visits for the same things, visits which seem to coincide with other family life-events.
2) Calling attention to rigid expectations which seem to be getting in the way, in spite of explanation aimed at clarifying the situation.
3) Calling attention to who is controlling the medical encounter: Who is making the decisions? Who is deciding which decisions are going to be decided? Who is deciding who decides? How has this been part of the problem?
4) Calling attention to issues of noncompliance, which have effectively undercut the doctor-patient contract: What has been involved in such behavior?

The solution to such dilemmas is usually closer when a broader perspective is applied. Another family member now appears to also be involved in noncompliant behavior. Deep-rooted views of a certain illness are seen to have exaggerated the patient's fears. It comes to light that the physician has been acting inappropriately to ward off certain feelings of his own.

When differences come up over the significance of the diagnosis, or over treatment, the physician is bound to investigate systemic issues further. He, after all, is the responsible party: the expert. The patient is sick, and has come to him for advice. The burden is on the physician.

The physician may pursue the pattern of interaction, thus initiating second-order change. Or he may look into his own feelings and his own (medical, family) system for contributing elements to the problem or unclarity. He may also look further into the patient's family or social system for clues to a deeper understanding: What are the patient's beliefs? What are the key people in his support system saying? What are his cultural and class norms? Are there any particular familial myths and images about this illness? ("I *know* it's my heart, doc—even though I'm only 28. Look, my Uncle John just died of a heart attack, and he was only 41. My Dad had a stroke when he was only 56. And now I got these horrible pains. . . . Can't you at least put me in the hospital for a few days . . . check me over . . . get some EKG's. . . ?")

Without delving into things more deeply, the physician runs a risk. If he simply pulls rank on a patient, forcing a diagnosis and/or plan without the patient's support, he deprives the patient of responsibility for his illness. Later, the patient may bridle at the physician's authoritarian manner and find another doctor if the diagnosis proves wrong. Alternatively, even if the diagnosis seems correct, the patient may subterraneanly sabotage treatment through noncompliance. Bypassing the diagnosis as a contract which involves the patient's agreeing at some level, then, invites problems and reflects a good deal of latent discord.

Thus, the diagnostic and treatment contract between the patient and physician, which is a *sine qua non* for effective management of the illness, requires delicate, continual negotiation, which needs to surmount many obstacles and conflicts to remain viable.

CHAPTER 12

The Contract Between the Physician and Members of the Family

Family members often become involved in issues around diagnosis and treatment. When someone in the family is sick, others want to know what's wrong, what caused it, how long their relative will be ill, and what they can do. Family support for a treatment program usually enhances the patient's cooperation and contributes to his or her improvement (Doherty and Baird, 1983; DiMatteo and DiNicola, 1982; Rosenbaum, 1983).

Families, however, are under constant stress, constantly changing to deal with new events and pressures in their lives. Normal developmental stages follow one upon the next: the couple has a baby; the baby becomes a toddler; another sibling is born; school begins; a member of the family falls sick or dies; and so on. Sudden illness or loss forces realignment of family forces. Crisis opens up in response to external events—Daddy loses his job—as well as to long accumulated internal strain—a young mother can no longer accept doing two loads of laundry, making the beds, cooking the meals, etc., every day, when she really wanted to be returning to work after the last baby was born.

Over time, different family members take on needed roles and responsibilities when a crisis, like an illness, arises. As different crises occur and the family grows older, these roles can be fought over, exchanged, shared, and relinquished. For years, for example, members of a family may have allowed Momma to make most family decisions on her own. But God forbid she should be hospitalized with a "condition"! Suddenly, children and grandchildren appear from all corners: the grandson doctor, the niece who is a nurse, the responsible younger brother. They will tell the physician secrets, and demand his own honest viewpoint. They may contest Momma's matriarchal role, especially if the illness is serious, and others may fight over the responsibility to make the decisions.

The physician tries to tell concerned family members what they need to know about their loved one's illness. Often, though, it is hard to figure out just who "the" responsible family member is, because a number of people are each claiming that role. At times, too, unaware of family bickering, the physician will "put his foot in it" and unwittingly side with one family faction against another. When the patient is elderly, when the prognosis is severe, when there is a question of mental incompetence or psychiatric illness, when children are involved, when in-laws are taking responsibility for their relatives, as well as on other occasions, the physician may be telling one thing to one family member and something else to the patient or to another family member.

When this happens, we can speak of different diagnostic contracts between physicians and different family members. These must always be viewed in relation to the family's hierarchical patterns, both overt and covert. Such contracts can actually create new hierarchies themselves, thus abolishing or sorely stressing the old ones. At times the situation can be even more complex: Different family members "enlist" or recruit different physicians, each of whom acts as an advocate of his or her faction's view.

Diagnoses in this sense can be *shared* with family members, *hidden* from them, given to them in somewhat *attenuated* form, given to them *instead of* to the patient, or given to them in different form than has been given to the patient. A few examples will bring out the intricacies involved.

Example 26

Essie L is a timid 76-year-old woman who somewhat resembles a frightened chicken. She is paranoid and fearful, always worrying someone will sneak out from under the bed or try to break through a window into her apartment. She comes into the office accompanied ("shepherded" might be a better term) by her sister Ida. Ida cares for her, helps her with her day-to-day chores, and makes sure her bills are paid. Ida also furtively gives her tranquilizer medication so she can sleep better and be less afraid.

Ida follows Essie into the office and helps her off with her coat. Essie blinks and smiles, slumping down in the examining chair. In the meantime, Ida winks and grimaces, waiting to catch my eye when Essie is not looking. Whatever Essie says, Ida qualifies it with a hidden wink or frown, a shake of the head or an "Oh God, do you hear the kind of things she's saying now!" expression. She makes silent syllables with her mouth: "No. She's lying. She's not taking her pills."

When Essie says that the neighborhood teenagers are trying to rape her, Ida shakes her head and taps her temples with an index finger to indicate that Essie is talking nonsense. When Essie starts mumbling her paranoid fantasies, Ida raises her eyebrows and shakes her head sadly.

According to Essie, she comes willingly to the physician, wanting to keep her blood pressure under control. According to Ida, Essie's visits have another purpose—so that the physician can follow Essie's deteriorating mental condition, prescribe appropriate medications, give Ida moral support in her difficult and unrewarding chore, and arrange for institutionalization should that become necessary.

Example 27

Mrs. M brings her teenage daughter to the doctor. "Tell him what's wrong," she says. "Nothing's wrong," the girl says. The mother exasperatedly turns to the doctor. "She's not eating," she says. "She got pains in her stomach." Then, turning back to the girl, angrily, "Tell him!" "It ain't nothing," the girl says, kicking at the side of the examining table and looking out the window as if she wanted to fly a million miles away, embarrassedly adolescent. "Hey," the doctor says. "What's going on? You say she's sick, and she says she isn't. What's going on? You both right, or what?" The mother looks as if she's going to choke someone. After all, she's dragged the kid to see the doctor, and now nothing's going right, and she's going to be made a fool and have to pay fifteen bucks for it as well. "Aw, she's always nagging at me," the girl says, leaping into the silence, testing the waters. . . .

Example 28

Mr. N's sister phones again. "I know you're going to see Billy at eleven," she says. "I just wanted to tell you . . . (heavy pause) . . . he's drinking again. I can't stop him. I'm scared he'll really hurt himself, or go out in the car and hurt someone else." She pauses.

"What do you want me to do?" the doctor says. "Whenever I talk to him, he says he isn't drinking much at all. Do you want to come in with him yourself and say what you're saying now?"

"No, I can't. He'd be furious." She pauses again, casting about for a solution. "But if you'd just put the fear o' God into him, he'll stop. I know he will. He stopped smoking when Dr. Martelli told him he had to. All you have to do is *scare* him."

"I don't believe in scaring patients," the doctor starts off, beginning to get irritated. "I mean, if he denies it, then . . ."

"You scare him," she repeats. "That's what Dr. Martelli did and it worked. But listen," she pauses again. "Don't say nothing to him about my calling."

"That's real hard for me to do . . ."

"Right, don't tell him I called. He wouldn't understand. You just scare him now. And thanks a lot, doc, thanks a lot."

Somehow, when the physician puts the receiver back on the hook, he feels as if he's been wrapped in some kind of sticky plastic, bound up, tied down, whatever you want to call it. "Triangulated" is too bland, too abstract a word to use. "Pushed to get stuck in the middle of a bad situation" sounds a lot better.

Many times, a "responsible family member" will negotiate with the physician, asking for the "truth" and trying to relay medical information to the rest of the family. This member, however, may not be at all objective, and she or he may often be embroiled in family conflict which has lasted for years. The family may even disagree over who the "responsible" member actually is.

Example 29

When Harriet P, an elderly black woman, became terminally ill and bed-ridden, she was cared for by her daughter. Day and night, this woman took care of her mother, sponge-bathed her, fed her, and tried to help her exercise. Finally, the woman weakened, and had to be hospitalized again. She was anemic and weak, and had developed pneumonia as well. The physician suggested nursing home care. "I just think it's too much for you to handle," he told the daughter. But the daughter refused. "No. I took care of her before, and I'll take care of her again," she said. "I want her to be sent back home with me."

However, Harry P, the woman's oldest son, visited the doctor in an angry mood. "Who does she think she is?" he growled. "I'm the oldest. *She* can't take care of my mother. Just look, she's right back in the hospital. That woman needs full-time nursing care. I think you should get her into one of the best of those nursing homes." "But just who is making the decision?" the physician asked. "I am," he answered. "I'm the oldest."

But when this "decision" was relayed to the patient's daughter, she was not convinced. "He doesn't do anything for her. How in hell can he make any decisions?" she said.

At times, the physician makes one kind of diagnostic contract with one family member and a different one with the patient. The "responsible" member may develop a good deal of guilt, too, over being unable to rescue or help her loved one, especially when the patient is a parent, and may then begin to argue interminably with the physician, members of the hospital staff, or other family members.

Example 30

Bob and Fannie Q came together to see the physician. They had been married for over 50 years, and now they had both grown ill. He had heart trouble and diabetes, and she had heart trouble and severe arthritis. In the past two years each had been hospitalized several times, and their health was deteriorating.

In recent months, the couple had come to the physician with their younger daughter Barbara. She took a keen interest in their health, and saw to it that they took their medications, followed their diets, and so on.

Unfortunately, Mr. Q grew worse. First he grew morose and depressed, and then his heart began to fail. His wife was hysterical, worried. He entered the hospital, saying he would never come out again alive, a prediction which he fulfilled.

In the period immediately after his death, Barbara continued to shepherd her mother to and from the doctor's office, on shopping trips, and to friends' homes. One day, however, she appeared in tears in the physician's office. Her older brother was now not talking to her; her older sister had spread rumors about her; and her "poor mother," distraught by the family squabbling, complained, "Oh God, why can't they be nice to one another?" and, in a fit of pique, promised to punish "all of them."

"Why me? Why *me*?" Barbara wept. "Haven't I been the one taking care of her? How can she be so ungrateful? I just can't take it anymore."

Patients and their families have a way of "triangulating" the doctor in order to avoid dealing with problems themselves. The physician becomes caught in the middle, asked to take sides in a family dispute.

Whichever way he chooses, he is damned; and the family will still go
through its own decision-making process. The only difference is that the
physician will now be cited as an authority by those whose position he
supports.

Other families may agree on the physician's position, but the physician
may not agree with them and may not want to do what they want him
to do. This becomes expressed as different views of what is wrong with
the patient.

Example 31

Michelle R, a ten-year-old girl, was constantly brought to the doctor
by her worried parents. This time, after three visits in four days,
they complained that the girl's sore throat was getting worse, that
her cough was deeper, and that "nothing is being done, nothing
is changing." When the doctor pointed out that throat cultures had
been negative twice, and that a long-lasting virus had been quite
prevalent in the community, they acknowledged the fact. Still, they
kept complaining that "something's got to be done."

"Do you want her in the hospital, then?" the doctor asked.

"Would it help?"

"Frankly, I don't think so. I think this is a virus, and it's just
going to take its course. We already gave her some antibiotics. I'd
rather see her at home, taking antibiotics and cough medicine, and
resting. . . ."

"Well," they hesitated. "Couldn't she get some extra treatment
in the hospital?"

"Yes. She might get some breathing treatments, blood tests . . ."

"Yeah . . . " they hesitated. "But we could do that at home with
a vaporizer."

"Right."

They paused again. "But we can't handle her at home. She's
getting worse and worse."

"What do you think is wrong with her?"

"I don't know. There's got to be something, 'cause she's not
getting any better, that's for sure."

It turns out that Michelle's mother, who worked the switchboard
at one of the local hospitals, did indeed want her in the hospital.
She would be able both to work and to look in on her daughter.
The more the physician tried to develop the diagnosis of a viral
upper respiratory infection, the more the family hemmed and
hawed and speculated on something else, something "really
wrong" with her.

The physician had no real choice, finally, but to admit the child. She was given cool mist and the same antibiotics as she had been on. She did well. The family was happy. Her benefits were terminated after three days, at which point she went home. The child was better. Both parents were grateful for the hospitalization and praised it for making Michelle well again and making sure nothing more serious was wrong.

In this instance, the family dynamics led to an unnecessary hospitalization. Unable to assuage the parents' anxiety, the physician was forced to admit their daughter, for he knew that she would be brought to the emergency room if he did not, and she would have been admitted from there.

There is another dimension to this story. This family had established a pattern with their previous physician, which encouraged frequent medical visits, even for very minor complaints, and fostered dependency on him for advice. Huygen and Smits (1983) have described the family doctor's role in somatically-fixated families, and this physician-family relationship fits their discussion well. Each tiny symptom is viewed as dangerous. Emotional distress in the family is rarely confronted openly; but, on the other hand, physical symptoms are accepted as a way of obtaining medical care.

At a deeper level, therefore, the physician's diagnosis of this situation might have read "upper respiratory infection in the youngest child of a somatically-oriented family." The family's own diagnosis of it was "severe bronchitis, possibly heading into pneumonia, requiring hospitalization."

It often happens, especially in a fee-for-service relationship, that patients who want some kind of procedure manage to get it. So long as they can find a doctor who accedes to their wishes, so long as emergency rooms continue to feed hungry hospitals, these people will be able to get what they want.

* * *

Another example of physicians' providing different diagnoses to different family members comes up around cancer or some other terminal illness. Family members usually plead that the patient "cannot take" the truth, and the physician must make a choice. Some physicians will respect these wishes; others will not. Some physicians naturally tend to keep painful truths from patients without being asked. Others categorically insist on "telling the truth." Whatever the style of physician and family, different diagnostic contracts are common in such situations, and lead to confusion if not handled with care.

Example 32

Harry S, a 67-year-old smoker, had experienced several episodes of bronchitis in a brief period of time. A hard worker, he had also devoted himself to caring for his wife, a good-hearted but quite portly woman, who was said to have been quite "fragile," having had two previous "nervous breakdowns." A year earlier, when he had prostate troubles, Mr. S had pleaded with his physician not to tell his wife if it turned out he had cancer. "She just wouldn't be able to cope with that kind of news," he said. "It would do her in." Now, once again, he repeated this request.

As it turned out, he had a fulminant form of lung cancer. His course was rapid and downhill. The physician had not told the true diagnosis to Mrs. S for several days, even though the truth of her husband's cancer seemed evident. One day, though, she cornered the physician in the hospital lounge and forced him to sit down. "Tell me the truth, now," she said. "Harry's got cancer, doesn't he? He's going to die."

"Yes," the physician said.

"I thought so," she replied, then paused for a long time, thinking deeply. "Well," she concluded, "I guess I had better start making arrangements for what has to be done, hadn't I?"

She bravely endured her husband's decline without crumbling, and was a strength to the rest of the family. Even today, though she weeps when she remembers him, she has borne up well, and his protective concern seems unwarranted.

Example 33

George T, a compulsive 70-year-old widower, developed a severe cough. X-rays showed a cancer. Consultation was obtained and a biopsy confirmed the diagnosis. He underwent resection of the lobe of the lung with tumor, and radiotherapy and chemotherapy followed.

"Am I cured?" he wanted to know.

"Tell him yes," the family urged. "You can't tell him the truth."

The physician confided the diagnosis of metastatic disease to the patient's children, but continued to hold out hope of a "curable tumor" to the patient.

Day after day, the patient weakened. But the physician continued to maintain that there was hope that his "congestion" would respond to treatment.

A rationale exists for establishing a different diagnosis with different family members. Investigation of patients' attributions of disease (Stoeckle and Barsky, 1980) has already been mentioned. People, responding to different class and cultural patterns, understand illness in different ways. Research into the evolution of people's conceptions of illness (Bibace and Walsh, 1981) shows that children pass through a sequence of stages in understanding illness. Some adults remain at "earlier" levels of understanding; further, it is common experience that many older or ill people regress psychologically to earlier ways of thinking. Thus, some adults feel that their disease is the result of some contagion, something they touched or breathed, or that it is a punishment for an evil or unthinking act, or that it is caused by some form of negligence.

Understanding this, it would be foolish to give the same explanation to each member of a family. The children might not understand the significance of the illness, and might be unnecessarily frightened, or blame themselves for a loved one's illness. Adults differ among one another psychologically, and understand the same "facts" differently. Thus, the "objective" physician who judiciously explains the diagnosis to everyone is usually explaining different things to each family member.

A variety of factors thus affects the diagnosis the physician will give to family members:

1) the actual diagnosis the physician makes to him/herself;
2) the severity of the illness and the risks it brings in its wake;
3) the patient's capacity to cope with the illness, as judged by the physician;
4) the family's capacity to cope with the illness, as judged by the physician;
5) what the family wants in the way of explanation from the physician;
6) other aspects of the patient's social support system;
7) the family dynamics, including the patient's family role and the role played by the illness;
8) the family's life stage and developmental tasks; and
9) the degree of responsibility the family members take on and care to pursue.

In sum, the contracts between physician and family members are varied and complex. Serving a variety of functions, they reflect both the family's dynamics and its interaction style. Looked at as a feature of the family system, not as the sole "property" of the identifiably ill member, the patient's illness may merit discussion with the entire family unit, probing which may help define the meaning of the illness, clarify how it fits into or runs contrary to the usual family patterns, assess the level of support the family can provide, and so on. Such a view runs counter to the customary organization of medical care, but it is sound and sensible, and might spare much suffering and confusion, as well as save money for those who pay the medical bill.

CHAPTER 13

The Contract Between Members of the Medical System

Other diagnoses involve agreements between members of the medical system—between two physicians, between a physician and others within the medical system, or between non-physicians. These are communications clarifying a patient's condition, so that people treating him or her can work more effectively together. This commonly occurs when a patient exhibits psychiatric symptoms or appears to be experiencing psychosomatic difficulties, or when the patient is a "difficult" management problem. It is a common feature in any referral process, and it inevitably happens when hospitalized patients are moribund.

Patients in pain often stimulate this process, with the staff's reaching a commonly shared diagnosis. Such patients may be felt to be exaggerating what they feel and are described as having "functional" pain, "supratentorial" pain, "hysterical" pain, and so on. When a physician makes this kind of diagnosis on the patient's chart, it is a signal that he thinks the patient's problem is mainly psychological. This can lead to the patient's being seen as someone without "real" pain, as hysterical, manipulative, faking, and so on—a view which will have dramatic consequences when the patient requests pain medication.

The diagnosis of a stress-related or "psychophysiological" disorder also says the physician thinks the patient is responding to an emotional stress, and that the illness is not "organic" but "functional." Such a diagnosis may be aimed at helping a consultant or the nursing staff by focusing attention on the emotional sources of the patient's suffering.

A woman with severe chest pain may be spared a potentially dangerous and costly workup if the diagnosis of a stress-related muscle pain is communicated to other physicians—for example, to the emergency room physicians or to the cardiology consultant. If a new physician sees her without contacting her family physician, he may hospitalize her in an intensive care unit, at great cost to herself and others, all in the name of "ruling out" an "organic" lesion.

On the other hand, such a diagnosis can be understood as calling the patient a "nut" or implying that he is willfully developing symptoms to get something from the physicians or staff. In this case, members of the medical system will be on guard against being "fooled" or "manipulated." The classification of a "psychosomatic" problem may thus disenfranchise the patient's complaints.

In light of recent legal rulings that patients have access to their records, communications among staff members in the hospital chart or via letters between consultant and referring physician can no longer be considered private matters, but may emerge as "damning" statements which split the patient from the physician, amid much anger and bitterness.

Example 34

Brenda U requested a gynecological consultation from her family physician. The family physician agreed, but in the referring letter made mention of the patient's "obvious neurotic personality." Miss U opened the letter and read it, then phoned her family physician in a state of outrage. She neither kept the referral appointment nor ever returned to the family physician.

CONTRACTS BETWEEN PHYSICIANS

Many disputes between one physician and another stem from different diagnostic views of the patient, views frequently grounded in the different perspectives each specialty pursues. Different specialists often vie with one another for control of the patient's case. These territoriality disputes touch issues of money and self-esteem. Diagnostic contracts between physicians often attempt to minimize such conflicts over how to manage the patient's illness.

Example 35

Arthur V had complained to his family doctor about joint pains, but his workup was negative. Not satisfied with his explanation,

Mr. V went to an orthopedic surgeon, and received a diagnosis of rheumatoid arthritis, which seemed to sit better with him. The family physician was angry, because there was no evidence for such a diagnosis; however, because of the orthopedist's status, he could not disagree openly. Consequently, he sent a note to the orthopedist explaining his own view that the patient had a form of "fibrositis" and asking his colleague to withhold further treatment for rheumatoid arthritis unless further evidence supported the diagnosis.

Example 36

Frances W complained of severe diarrhea and abdominal cramps. The treating physician diagnosed the problem as a severe irritable bowel syndrome, but Ms. W wanted further consultation. The gastroenterologist chosen began an elaborate "organic" workup to exclude diseases of the small and large bowel, etc. When the evaluation turned up nothing, the consultant wrote a note in the chart agreeing with the earlier diagnosis, and thus closing the door on the patient's search for an organic source of her distress.

Example 37

Karen X, an elderly widow, worried a great deal about her heart. She felt it was failing. Although she did indeed have a cardiac condition, her family physician felt it was not as pressing a problem as was her worry over it. She asked for a referral to a cardiologist, who recommended a variety of new medicines and spoke about the possibility of cardiac catheterization. Mrs. X was staunchly set against surgery, but she interpreted the cardiologist's medicines and suggestions as proof that her cardiac condition was very, very bad, and that she was about to die. The family physician shared his perspective with the cardiologist. The latter said he was just carrying through his understanding of the referral. But after the talk, the two of them agreed not to begin any new medicines or mention any more procedures, but simply to manage the patient as she had been managed before, trying to control her worry which, they now agreed, presented the main management problem.

Physical symptoms of depression are another common problem in family practice. In such cases, patients fi quently deny the underlying feelings which promote the symptoms, thereby making treatment quite difficult. When they fall into the hands of a somatically-oriented specialist, the physicalization of their symptoms may be locked in unless the latter perceives what is going on at a deeper level.

Physicians need not always disagree, of course. Much of the time, they will agree about a patient's diagnosis. It occasionally happens, however, that the patient does not know about this, or disagrees.

In most instances, treating physicians discuss the patient's condition with the consultants they call in for assistance. The doctors may talk together in the hospital corridor, the doctors' station, or in the lounge. They may "touch base" by telephone. Through such communication, they "get their signals straight" and reach a common diagnostic and therapeutic opinion, which can then be transmitted uniformly to the patient and his or her family. At times, however, they do not agree. They may have genuine differences of opinion about the patient's condition. They may actually be competing for control of the patient's treatment, as happens increasingly today when specialists take charge of the patient for their own particular procedures, while the generalist is relegated to the background (this has also led the specialist to wind up providing post-crisis continuing care, which in some instances leads to accusations of "stealing the patient"). The recent push to limit the number of physicians who can care for a hospitalized patient—through insurance companies' rejecting claims for "duplicate services"— means that generalists often have to hand over the temporary care of their patients to some specialist, and then have to watch while procedures with which they disagree are carried out. This can happen when a patient is placed on a teaching service, whose medical students or residents are eager to pursue every problem the patient may have, thereby ordering (what appear to the generalist to be) unnecessary tests. It may arise when a patient is sent to another hospital, out of reach of the family doctor, or when patients come to Emergency Rooms for help. It may happen when the family physician simply loses legal control of the patient's case.

Example 38

Joshua Y came to the emergency room complaining of a cold and crampy leg. He was admitted by the house officer to a vascular surgeon, who ordered arteriograms on the patient and suggested surgery. The patient's family physician had no access to his management, except as a consultant himself. He disagreed with plans for surgery, feeling that the patient's cardiac status was shaky, but was helpless to stop the operation. The patient developed cardiac troubles during the operation and subsequently died.

CONTRACTS BETWEEN PHYSICIANS AND OTHER MEDICAL PERSONNEL

Anyone who has worked in a hospital or large medical office knows that staff conflicts are common, especially around patients whose diagnoses are unclear. For example, disputes between attending physicians and the nursing staff on an inpatient hospital ward often occur and can expand to include other personnel: consultants, emergency room personnel, and social workers. When nurses disagree with the patient's physician, they may organize support from other health workers in order to isolate the physician. Such combined pressure may force the physician to change his or her ways. Often, too, patients are "triangulated" into this dispute: they complain of being treated poorly by the staff; the staff blames the physicians for their patients' "difficult" behavior; physicians side with their patients and criticize the nurses. The nurses claim that the physicians' difficult patients reflect their own difficult personality, or that their patients are manipulating them.

Physicians may only see their patients for a few minutes a day, but they make much more money than the nurses, and give them orders which they must carry out. In the meantime, the nurses have to take care of patients' daily needs, and minister to a large number of patients as well, often without adequate coverage. Their allegiance is to the rules of the hospital and to the other hospital workers. Physicians' unpredictable capacity to disregard hospital rules, combined with their often haughty attitude, can contribute to bitter disputes.

Example 39

Artie Z, a middle-aged diabetic man, complained about severe pains in his legs. He felt they came from his diabetes and often demanded analgesics for them, claiming that no one else could know how badly he hurt. His physician felt that the neurological and vascular complications of diabetes might well be contributing to his pains, but he sensed the presence of many psychosocial factors as well.

The nursing staff of the hospital saw Mr. Z as a drug addict. They did not believe he had pain, and they managed to make him wait for his medication beyond the point when it was supposed to be given. This drove him wild with frustration. They responded that it was not their fault, because they were understaffed.

The physician tried to explain the situation to the head nurse, and finally the two of them reached an understanding of Mr. Z's pain problem. But the younger nurses on the floor rejected this view, still claiming that the physician was giving too much medication to the patient.

When the night nurse refused to give Mr. Z his medication one evening, claiming that he had asked for it 15 minutes too soon, the patient became agitated, tried to climb out of bed, fell, and broke his hip. The staff wrote its own accident report, which disagreed sharply with Mr. Z's own version of the incident. There were mutual accusations. The nurses defended one another. Mr. Z tried to sign out of the hospital.

The concern with how "aggressive" one should be in pursuing a patient's illness often arises between physicians and the nursing staff. One example of this involves the "No Code" orders that say a moribund patient should not be revived in case of cardiac arrest. Others involve how energetically to treat a urinary infection in a patient with a catheter; whether or not to catheterize incontinent patients; and whether sleeping pills can be given at the same time as pain pills.

Disputes can break out between physician and social workers, too. For example, the physician may feel that an elderly patient needs social support and sedative medication, and that this is a task for the Social Service Department in the hospital. But the social worker may decline such a request, fearing that the patient is really suffering from some severe medical condition, which the physician is not adequately investigating. Thus, each of them may feel the other is "passing the buck" and not looking to cope with the patient's condition.

Social workers may also sometimes feel that the physician is dumping his or her patient on the hospital. This view follows from their particular perspective (hospital employee; competing professional) and can lead to angry infighting over the "disposition" of an elderly patient—home, nursing home, a relative's home, continued hospitalization, and so on.

The "team" approach to patient-care, often talked about but less often pursued, holds that each member of the medical-care team is important and merits the others' respect. Because disputes usually wind up affecting the patient's health, agreement on a diagnostic and treatment contract between disagreeing members of the "team" is critical. Without such a contract, each medical-care group tends to struggle for control with the others. Moreover, some patients thrive in such an atmosphere, setting the healers against one another ("Let's you and him fight") or accusing everyone of being incompetent or uncaring ("Doesn't anybody love me?"). In truth, however, no one benefits from such a situation.

CONTRACTS BETWEEN NON-PHYSICIANS

Hospital staff frequently meet together to discuss the patients. At such meetings, agreements are made about the diagnosis and treatment plan of a number of patients, which differ from what the physician may have laid forth. As we shall see in the next chapter, however, such agreements may lay the basis for how a patient will be perceived and treated throughout the hospital stay.

CHAPTER 14

The Contract Between a Patient or Family Member and a Non-Physician Member of the Medical System

Once the medical and family systems have been drawn out, the combinations of diagnostic contracts appear almost endless. The expansion of modern medical technology has brought patients and their families into contact with a variety of non-physician health-care workers, any one of whom may directly influence a diagnostic decision. When these "paraprofessionals" become expert in their own particular area of the health-care world, new possibilities emerge for enhancing or undercutting the integrated care of the patient's problem. In particular, rivalries with the treating physician may emerge which affect the overall care of the patient.

Example 40

Linda A was an elderly woman with severe lung disease. She needed home oxygen and almost daily home chest therapy. Her therapist reported directly to the hospital Chief of Pulmonary Medicine, but not to the family physician whose patient Ms. A had been for many years. Thus, when the therapist found the patient more short of breath than usual, he phoned the Chief and brought the patient to the hospital for him to examine. In fact, he believed Ms. A's family physician had but a minimal grasp of pulmonary medicine, and he felt he was doing the best thing for her by bringing her to the hospital.

The family physician, who had known Ms. A for years, would have preferred to deal with her problem himself, outside of the hospital. Furthermore, feeling familiar with the basics of pulmonary medicine himself, he felt competent to treat his patient should she require hospitalization, short of the intensive care unit. At the very least, he expected to be notified of her course.

The respiratory therapist's diagnosis that the patient's condition had severely deteriorated, however, made Ms. A think her own physician did not understand her problem. She had shared the therapist's respect for the pulmonary specialist; so, when he said she should be hospitalized, she entered the hospital as the latter's patient. Because she did not have enough money for two physicians and because she felt that her main problem was her lung disease, she decided to leave the generalist and become one of the pulmonary specialist's patients.

The contract between therapist and the patient thus led to a dissolution of one doctor-patient relationship and the start of another. The latter, however, emphasized hospital-based care to a much higher degree than had her earlier one. This had major consequences: First, the cost of the patient's care increased; second, the lack of an integrated whole-person approach to her problems led her to focus exclusively on her respiratory difficulty. In choosing to do this, she was able to deny other, equally important psychosocial issues, such as her recently being widowed and her steady loss of close friendships and ensuing social isolation. Choosing to see herself as a pulmonary patient suited her view of herself as a total "victim" and reinforced her drawing away from others who had cared for her. The pulmonary specialist was not interested in exploring this dimension of his patient's situation.

Example 41

Marian B, a 45-year-old married woman, was hospitalized for evaluation of a breast lump. The lump turned out to be cancerous, and she had to have the breast removed. Her family physician was a support throughout the ordeal, and the surgeon was kind and considerate. Yet neither of them could deal with the many issues in her mind, issues which were raised by the spectre of being deformed, by the thought of cancer in the other breast, and by the parallel Ms. B now felt with her mother, who had also had breast cancer. One of the nurses on the floor, however, began to spend a good deal of time with her. She had had breast cancer, too, six years earlier. Ms. B felt this woman, close to her own age, understood what she was feeling and could answer her questions. The meaning and significance of her own illness were developed through daily long conversations with this nurse. Afterwards, she looked back on the nurse as the most important person to her through the whole illness experience.

Example 42

Hilda C was very upset when she came to her physician. Her jaw hurt, and she didn't know why. Finding nothing abnormal, the physician ordered an X-ray at the local hospital. The X-ray technician, after taking the pictures, made a pained grimace. When the patient asked what was wrong, the technician said, "Well, I think your jaw is displaced. Have you been in an accident lately?"

Ms. C was a person who tended to become hysterical at the drop of a hat. After being told that her jaw was dislocated, she called her doctor frantically, relaying what the technician had said. At her own request ("No," she said. "I can't wait until tomorrow!"), she was scheduled for an immediate specialist consultation.

When the oral surgeon examined her, he felt the only problem was her dentures. The "official" X-ray report came back as "normal." Yet the technician's contract with this patient had led her to extreme anxiety, an unnecessary consultation, and some loss of confidence in her own physician who, after all, had scheduled the consultation.

Example 43

Jeb D was upset over his mother's illness. He didn't understand what had caused it, and he didn't understand what it meant. His mother's doctor didn't take time to explain the situation to him either, and he always seemed too hurried. One afternoon, however, when he was visiting his mother, the man who cleaned and polished the hospital floors stopped by to talk. His mother had suffered from the same problem, and he said he "just wanted to say hello" to Mr. D and chat for a few minutes. Mr. D quickly warmed to the man, and the two of them spent an hour talking. "I got more from that man today," he said to his wife, "than I got from that Dr. N all week."

Other similar agreements can take place—for example, over the phone between a patient and the doctor's receptionist; between the visiting nurse and an elderly patient's daughter ("Well, I think she's retaining fluid. Maybe you should speak to her doctor about prescribing a diuretic."); between the dietician and the patient's husband ("This kind of diabetes is very hard to control. You'll have to pay careful attention. . . ."), and so on. The general principle is that anyone who is part of the medical system, and who is therefore stamped with the emblem of "medical expert," can establish a diagnostic contract with the patient or any member of his family.

This having been understood, it is clear that the possibilities for conflict and misunderstanding around any serious illness, as well as for beneficial contact, warmth, and support, are tremendous.

CHAPTER 15

Contracts Between a Physician and a Third Party

Another category of diagnosis includes occasions when physicians are asked to provide expert opinion about their patient to a third party. In this group are physicians' letters to welfare departments, the courts, insurance companies, employers, schools, disability, social security, and other public agencies. Usually, such statements ask the physician to give the patient's medical diagnosis, its causal relation to some accident, occupational injury, or exposure to work-related hazard, the degree of disability, and the estimated time when the patient might return to work. Such interchanges deal with what Parsons (1951) discussed under the patient's "sick" role.

Such requests cascade upon the practicing physician from a variety of sources. Patients claim they cannot pay their gas bill because of illness. They want a special subway pass, handicapped license plates, a certificate to stay out of work. They want documents for court procedures, letters for a lawyer, and statements for disability appeals. The physician is asked to certify that the patient's home oxygen is necessary for survival, or else the oxygen company will not bring it. In today's society, physicians have become an ultimate authority on people's capacity to work. They are the legitimizers, the arbitrators of disability, the excuse-givers: A's absence from school or work was due to illness; B is in good physical shape and can work or play hockey; C has no communicable disease; D is too ill for jury duty; E needs a homemaker; F needs Meals on Wheels; G needs home nursing care.

Such requests drag physicians beyond the usual doctor-patient relationship, for they are being asked to serve someone else's interests, not theirs or the patient's. Indeed, such requests often put physicians in a bind: As the patient's sympathetic confidant, they may have taken on the role of ombudsmen vis-à-vis public agencies. Now, suddenly, they are being asked for an "objective" report from these same agencies, who will then decide the patient's degree of incapacity, a decision which will affect the patient for the rest of his or her life.

At times, too, physicians are asked to serve the interests of the state: the public good. They may be required to give evidence of venereal or other contagious disease, report suspected child abuse, and tell authorities about possible drug abuse.

The question is, whose interests do physicians serve, and when? Do physicians always serve the one who pays their bills? If so, do they then serve the patient when the patient pays and the state or the insurance company when the latter commissions their services? If so, what then happens to their professional judgment? When do physicians simply serve the interests of "medical truth?" Sometimes the patient begs the physician to distort the truth ("I'll lose my Medicaid if you say I can work!"), and sometimes the state urges him or her to take its side ("Please answer the following three questions about your patient's alleged disability. . . ."). Furthermore, when the physician is asked to describe a patient's diagnosis, what level of diagnosis is appropriate to relate?

The physician's allegiance may be torn between his deepest conviction, his duty to society, his responsibility to whoever is employing him, and his relationship to the patient and the patient's family. Traditionally, it has been assumed, as Waitzkin and Waterman (1976) make clear, that physicians "impartially" serve the dominant class interests of their society. Thus, they can be trusted to tell the truth to the courts, not to give welfare certificates out indiscriminately, and to weed out moral slouchers from the ranks of the truly sick. However, the recent view of physicians (especially the family physician) as the patient's advocate appears to challenge this.

Frequently, physicians who owe no allegiance to the patient can be relied on to serve the interests of those who employ them. Examples of this can be found among physicians on disability boards, company doctors, "experts" who give testimony for different sides in a court case, doctors, and so on.

Example 44

A company physician who had held his position for 15 years asked
another physician to take care of sick call while he was on vacation.
Before he left, he encouraged his colleague to spend some time
with Marty, the company's president, who was supposed to be a
"great guy."

The younger physician found sick call quite interesting, especially as many of the workers had obvious occupationally-related
illnesses, the most frequent being a tendonitis caused by repetitive
assembly-line work. The physician prescribed medications for such
complaints, as well as the usual course of treatment: 7-10 days of
rest away from the physical strain which had caused the problem.

When the older physician returned, he quickly buttonholed his
colleague. "Hey, you did a good job," he said. "Of course, maybe
you could have spent a little more time with Marty." (The younger
man's only contact with this fatuous gentleman had been when he
stuck his head in the office to ask for free samples of an antihypertensive medication.) "Except for one thing . . ." He paused
and drew the younger man closer, arm around his shoulder in a
confidential gesture. "You've got to watch out for these workers.
They're the lowest of the low. Lucky to have the job." He made
a sour, distasteful face. "Working for three dollars an hour, the
lowest of the low. You give 'em an inch, and they'll take a mile.
You know what I mean?"

"Not exactly."

"Look," he said. "When they come in with some complaint or
another, you don't want to give 'em so much time off. They'll just
piss it away anyway. Give 'em a few pills, maybe a day or two out
of work at the most. And leave it at that."

It was clear where this company physician's allegiance lay.

Such attitudes are no secret to patients who move from one physician
to another in an attempt to find someone who will "listen to their side
of the story." They are widespread, and explain why disability boards,
insurance physicians, and welfare physicians predictably offer up adverse judgments regarding patients' capacity to work.

When the city government, for example, pays a physician to determine
a claimant's degree of cardiac disability for retirement reasons, it puts
him into a very different relationship to the patient than as the patient's
own physician.

Example 45

Five years ago, a physician had told Manny E, a 58-year-old fireman, that he had "horrible angina" and would be lucky to live another two years. Following a normal stress test, he had gone for cardiac catheterization and, according to him, had "almost died on the table." For the next two years, he lived in a state of panic.

Whenever he became upset, he developed chest pains. His face was transformed into a mask of depression, suffering, and tension. His wife felt certain he was going to bring on a heart attack. After several years of worry over his "heart condition," he concluded that he would have to retire. He spoke to his boss who, he said, told him, "Okay. Just get a doctor's note, and we'll put it through." After all, after 25 years on the job he deserved some consideration.

His family doctor wrote a simple note saying Mr. E had been treated for angina pectoris for years. But as it turned out, the note was not enough. The Fire Department authorities sent the patient for further tests with a cardiologist, a specialist whom the city paid for his services. This physician examined Mr. E and scheduled further tests. The patient refused. "Hey," he angrily explained. "I got my own doctor, whom I trust with all my heart. What do I need other tests for? If my doctor felt I should have other tests, he'd order them. Right? Remember, I almost *died* the last time I had stress tests and scans and all that. In fact, there was a guy in bed next to me who *did* die. So, no thanks. I ain't taking any more tests. Just put my papers through."

The cardiologist said that, without the requested tests, he wouldn't have enough information to process the retirement papers. This was especially true since the tests done five years ago, according to him, had been normal. "What do you mean, *normal*," Mr. E cried. "That ain't what they told me *then*. And if they were normal, how come I got these pains all the time?"

The patient refused any further tests. At this point, his superiors threatened not to grant his disability. They said he could take an early retirement if he wanted, which carried a lower pension than disability, and they hinted that if he refused to take it and continued to refuse the cardiologist's tests, they might have to call him back to work. Refusing that, he could be fired, and would then be out of work with no pension at all.

He refused everything. Sticking by his guns, he demanded that the case be presented to the Board as it was.

The Retirement Board asked for statements from three physicians: an expert employed by the Board, the cardiologist, and Mr. E's own physician. The family physician was asked to answer the question, "Is there any medical evidence or information which could document that the claimant did *not* have the problem he said he had?" "No, of course not," the physician answered. He submitted a full description of his years of contact with the fireman.

The Chairman of the Medical Panel was the Board's own medical expert. In a display of understanding that, rivaling Solomon, cut to the core of the matter, he declared that the patient was indeed entitled to his retirement. He wrote:

> If I was his doctor, I would urge him to have such studies (as the cardiologist requested), if only to help allay his severe anxiety, regarding the diagnosis of heart disease that has been made in good faith by his doctors. However, I do not believe it is the function of a medical panel in a retirement case to demand that a claimant have such an exhaustive and expensive study either at the Board's or the claimant's expense, in order that action be taken by the Board. In this case I have the choice of either refusing to pursue the matter further unless such studies are carried out, of approving, or of disapproving the claim. In the case of Mr. E, the clinical symptoms are suggestive of angina pectoris due to heart disease, and he has been diagnosed and treated in good faith as a cardiac patient by his doctors. He has a severe and persistent anxiety reaction regarding his condition and this would continue, I believe, if he continued to work, and he would be unfit to perform all of the duties of a firefighter. I am therefore approving this application on the basis of the clinical diagnosis and treatment. If the Board sees fit to take another stand, they should do so.

Many other applicants are not so fortunate as Mr. E.

* * *

It is a familiar dilemma. The patient becomes trapped between the medical system and another bureaucracy, which has control over his life. Important decisions hang in the balance. If the medical system serves the patient's interests, one kind of report will be written. If the physician's report serves the interests of those paying the bill, another report will come down.

Waitzkin and Stoeckle (1976) have discussed the role of physicians in transmitting society's dominant values. Physicians not only "transmit" these values; they also act vigorously on them themselves. Their values shape how they deal with their patients' suffering, and explain why patients often feel "stonewalled." Their doctor doesn't seem to understand what they are saying. Their doctor doesn't understand what is at stake when they ask for a simple letter, excuse, or certification. Patients' feelings are often accurate. Society has placed physicians in a critical, powerful position, controlling access to a number of health-related services, knowing that they can be trusted not to give out too many excuses.

Other examples of diagnosis as a contract between physicians and third parties are:

1) The use of psychiatric testimony to determine if a person "knew the difference between right and wrong" at the time of a criminal act. If the person did, he can be tried for his crimes. If not, he has been relieved of responsibility for it by an "insanity defense."
2) The use of expert testimony to establish the degree of disability resulting from an accident or injury. If such disability is established, the claimant may be entitled to disability payments, compensation, or other benefits. If not, the claimant will have to find other sources of income and reimbursement for medical payments, living costs, and lost income.
3) The use of the physician to establish eligibility for a number of free services offered by the community to those either ill and unable to pay, or simply disabled in some way by illness. Examples of this are welfare payments given to those too sick to work; free transportation to and from physicians' offices and hospitals; free meals; free homemaker services or other forms of at-home therapy; free medicines and medical equipment (oxygen tanks, hospital beds, wheelchairs).
4) The use of the physician to declare *ineligibility* for some tasks: jury duty, gainful occupation, and the like.

If diagnostic certainty could be obtained, the appeal to physicians for data in eligibility or disability determinations might have a sounder basis. But since many diagnostic impressions are hypotheses at best, the prestige of the physician's statement conceals the fact that it is mainly opinion.

SUMMARY

This discussion of diagnosis as a social contract has attempted to clarify some problems around diagnosis that emerge in practice. Diagnostic contracts are created by mutual consent. They are affected by social roles and expectations, and may be formed between many different people involved around the illness. Conflicting contracts may exist simultaneously. Biomedical "facts" may be qualified, distorted, or denied in arriving at some of these contracts. An unclear world, in which any number of diagnostic contracts compete for dominance, calls for careful, sensitive management of the patient's illness in its total context.

Part III
Nosological and Other Questions

CHAPTER 16

Nosology and Classification

Any discussion of diagnosis should examine the schemes by which illnesses are named and grouped. This falls under the purview of nosology, the branch of medicine which deals with the classification of diseases. Nosology had remained stagnant for many years, but it is now developing new life amid growing controversy (cf. Hyde, 1983).

The perspective I have put forward would argue that a contemporary nosology should describe both the biomedical and the psychosocial factors surrounding any particular illness. Its terminology should situate illness in context, and be able to guide epidemiological studies of illness and the family.

No such nosology exists today.

If it did, what would the tasks of such a nosology be?

A classification system of illness has three basic tasks:

1) scientific: to further the development of knowledge through study of the natural history of disease;
2) clinical: to guide treatment and therapy of particular problems; and
3) economic: to enable health professionals to get paid for their work.

Diseases can be thought of as clearly discrete static entities or as dynamic processes with differing degrees of expression. Feinstein (1967) accepts the latter view when he uses Venn diagrams to describe the different statistical distribution of the possible signs and symptoms of a given disease process. Following this model, diseases appear as clumps of symptoms, with different probabilities of mortality and morbidity. This model does indeed fit the clinical facts more closely: A given illness can present in different ways. It can run different courses. It can respond differently to treatment in two individuals.

Not all heart attacks, for example, present with chest pain. Some present with epigastric distress; some with shoulder pain; some are clinically "silent." Some illnesses can be diagnosed by a lab test, but may not produce any clinical symptoms (myeloma in its early stages). Other illnesses can be discovered only by a physical exam, not by any lab tests; they too may produce no clinical distress (hypertension). Still other illnesses may be diagnosed only by their clinical picture and response to treatment, and there may be no known lab test or physical measurement for their diagnosis (tension headaches). Some cases of a disease have greater, some lesser, degrees of systemic involvement (rheumatoid arthritis). The discovery of the same disease in two individuals may be followed by death within six months in one, and life for another decade in the other. And so it goes, with marked variation in disease penetration, expression, and morbidity.

Ideally, nosology should provide a scheme capable of encompassing whatever physicians understand about illness. But different physicians understand things differently, and they may rank the factors affecting illness in different hierarchies. This can make nosology mean different things for different people, and gives rise to controversy. Those preferring a narrow focus on biomedical factors will want a nosology to reflect advances in biochemistry, cellular physiology, and immunology. Those who prefer a broader perspective will want a nosology to describe illness in its full psychosocial context. Those interested in a systems approach may well want both.

Any proposed nosology must take on the dominant controversy in the field. At the current time, this revolves around taking the family as a basic unit of medical care.

THE FAMILY AS A UNIT OF MEDICAL CARE

There has been much controversy, especially in family practice, over whether the individual or the family is the basic "unit of medical care." If it is the former, then a nosology has little reason to pursue the family dimensions of illness, except as they may clarify an individual's sickness.

If, on the other hand, the family is seen as a legitimate unit of care, then a family-oriented nosology becomes appropriate—in fact, imperative. One cannot otherwise describe the sicknesses that emerge in family systems.

The dispute is a variation on the familiar argument between "narrow" and "broad" points of view, between biomedical and biopsychosocial models. But the outcome of a struggle over nosology has profound implications for both medical education and medical practice. It will determine how physicians are trained to view their field, how patients think about their illnesses, and how insurance carriers reimburse health-care providers for their work.

Today, no standard diagnostic code views illness from a family perspective. No standard "service" codes describe treatment for family—as opposed to individual—problems.* The physician who understands his or her patients' problems in a broader context—i.e., family turmoil in the context of the impending death of a matriarch who has dominated the family for five decades, presenting as one son's chest pain, a daughter's back pain, a granddaughter's migraines—must often use some other diagnosis in order to be reimbursed by most "third-party" payers.

Therapists, too, may have to bill for treating a single family member's "depression," even if the treatment is family therapy. The family physician may have to bill for treating "hypertension," even though the treatment may have been conjoint counseling with both the hypertensive patient and his wife, in the conviction that the couple's turmoil was exacerbating the husband's hypertension. "Manufacturing" diagnoses this way, however, is time-consuming, aggravating, and feels inherently dishonest. It also keeps everyone focused more closely on the biomedical model, and thus makes it harder to create new diagnostic codes which can legitimize family diagnostic entities and family-oriented services.

If medical or therapy services for family-related problems are not reimbursable, few physicians will provide them.

Some family physicians have already raised this issue. Lee Hyde is designing a nosology which can incorporate family-centered problems, integrating family problems into the currently used ICD-9 classification (unpublished manuscript, 1984). Such a revision would let the interested family doctor identify, diagnose, and treat family medical problems, as well as individual patients' sicknesses.

---

*Psychotherapy is an exception. It does have codes which embrace both couple and family work, but these codes remain in the therapist's domain and cannot be used, except with much "stretching the point," by others.

This very concept, however, raises questions: In what sense can the family be considered a *unit of care* in medicine?

The advocates of family diagnosis make a simple case. People's problems, both medical and emotional, are better understood and more effectively treated when viewed in their psychosocial—especially their family—context. The family physician, who sees people in such a context regularly, understands how one person's illness can affect other family members, and how illness often emerges in one family member after a period of shared stress and turmoil. The family physician observes varied effects of illness in the family—snowballing, ricocheting, grouping, scapegoating—and how illness affects successive generations, or how a single stressful event simultaneously affects several family members.

Primary-care physicians counsel patients at times of family stress and treat many stress-related (psychosomatic) illnesses. Such activity naturally fits into a more all-encompassing nosology.

Our earlier discussion of the relationship between illness and the family documented many ways psychosocial (especially family) factors influence illness. Advocating the family as a basic unit of medical care gives a way to apply this information. A problem arises, however, over differences about "how far" this metaphor should be applied. Some advocates of the "family as a basic unit of care" view go beyond viewing individual patients in their family context. They even go beyond viewing the interacting family members as a dynamic system, with its own rules. Sometimes it appears that the systems thinkers go so far as to claim the existence of a family system with its own independent "dysfunction" and "pathology." Such a "unit" becomes an object of care in its own right.

These views have attracted much debate (cf. Carmichael, 1983; Ransom, 1983a, b, c).

The essential argument against the broader view rests on the conviction that only individuals can be patients. This view respects the unique qualities of the doctor-patient relationship, especially its privacy, and extols what the Carmichaels have called (1981) "the relational model" in family practice. It holds that, no matter how critically important familial (or other) factors may be in the course of anyone's illness, the physician has no license to impose patients' families on the treatment of their illness. Of course, if the patient wishes it, his or her relatives can be involved—but not automatically.

Carmichael (1983) points out that physicians usually treat patients one by one, that only rarely are *all* members of a single family seen by one family doctor, and that families extend far beyond the nuclear family into social networks which cannot be objects of medical care, even though they affect the individual patient's health. While he approves of efforts to see patients in their social context, he asserts that the basic relationship is still between physician and family.

Ransom, responding to this argument, points out that the physician is frequently asked to consider the well-being of others in the patient's family circle. Contagious diseases, psychotic behavior, nervous disorders, and many disabling illnesses come to mind as ready examples of what he means. Agreeing with Carmichael's concern with the relational aspects of family practice, Ransom criticizes him for shutting the door on a promising avenue of research and interest, by denying the legitimacy of focus on the family. The debate, of course, continues.

Carmichael respects the relationship at the heart of medicine. But he caricatures the view he opposes. No one advocates "imposing" a patient's family on his illness. Rather, one simply has to recognize whatever "family" exists. Physicians have to expand their horizons. They have to accept the importance of the patient's family: inquire about the family, be sensitive to family members' requests, and struggle to situate the patient's life problems in its own world. At times, for example, a couple will come to the physician complaining they cannot work out their marriage alone. An entire family can go through crisis at the loss of a parent and may request a chance to talk it through. A child with asthma or severe neurodermatitis may not be treatable unless the physician delves into the parents' relationship.

Therapists have already begun looking into the relationship between family dynamics and illness, but most physicians act as if their work does not exist. If the family unit is, however, a meaningful and relevant entity, then physicians must delve into it. Understanding cannot be held back by plunging one's head into the sand.

Surely, one can respect individual patients' integrity without simultaneously denying the existence of larger possible treatment units. The entire field of epidemiology rests upon such a broader perspective. If a strep throat can travel from one family member to another, what is to be said about the effects of a father's alcoholism or a mother's suddenly catastrophic illness on others in the family milieu?

Huygen's excellent monograph (1982) speaks convincingly to this objection. He points out several common familial patterns of illness and outlines the effects of family crisis on members other than the identified patient. For example, he speaks about the family whose mother or father dies, the family with a chronically ill parent, the family with a handicapped child, and the family which "needs" a chronic patient.

In addition, normal stages of family development are often times of increased medical or psychological symptoms. Nodal points, times of change, the times of the birth of a child, the departure of a teenager, the death of a family member, etc., can be occasions for the outbreak of both what can be termed illness behavior and dysfunctional psychosocial behavior. Family problems often run along a different time and space "axis" than do their members' medical problems, and thus they cannot be comprehended by simply adding up the individual members' diagnoses. Extending this understanding to the interplay between socioeconomic and political factors and illness—as, say, in the case of war, famine, inflation, widespread unemployment, flood, and so on—can provide a way of understanding widespread "ripple" or "wave" phenomena in the appearance of certain medical or psychiatric processes.

Much can be said, then, for extending the notion of diagnosis to involve at least the family unit, and perhaps more. As to whether all families can be (or should be) diagnosed, we will address that question later.

DIAGNOSIS AND PAYMENT

Increasingly today, physicians contract diagnoses with insurance carriers and the state (Blue Cross and Blue Shield, Medicaid, Medicare, and so on) in order to be paid. If their diagnosis does not follow a reimbursable code, however, there will be no payment. This means physicians must currently follow the established codes, codes which are dominated by the biomedical model and which promote a focus on the individual, not the family, and on the organ system, not on the whole person.

Current diagnostic and procedural codes present more obstacles than their lack of family diagnoses. For example, current codes reward technical and surgical procedures more than they do procedures which involve sitting and talking to a patient or a family. (An EKG taken in five minutes in the office may bring $45. A half-hour spent talking and listening may not even be reimbursable.) In other words, time spent in an interpersonal, give-and-take manner has less value than time spent doing procedures. Technology is more highly prized than the interpersonal contact which is supposed to be the basis of the doctor-patient relationship.

Revising the diagnostic codes to include terms covering family-oriented problems may be inadequate unless one also works to equalize the "procedural" codes. Such equalization would give more importance to preventive medicine, yearly checkups, counseling sessions, patient education, and so on.

For example, emergency room visits are currently reimbursed lucratively. This is because they are supposed to be for acute, emergency care. (By definition, of course, any problem treated in an emergency room is an "emergency" and its care will be reimbursed by insurance carriers as such.) But a sore throat is the same whether seen in a physician's office, in an EmergiCenter walk-in clinic, or in a hospital emergency room. So is a bad headache. Yet insurance policies frequently cover any kind of treatment, including routine medical care, when it is provided in the emergency room, but refuse to cover such care provided (for a quarter the cost) in a family physician's office.

Knowing this, patients may prefer being seen for free (even though it costs their insurance company dozens of dollars more), rather than paying $15. or $20. out of their own pockets. In this case, the place where services are rendered actually "diagnoses" the medical condition which is treated there.

The absence of family-oriented diagnostic codes and the existence of a sharp differential which rewards technology and "biomedicine" are factors, then, which link nosology and payment.

CHAPTER 17

Attempts at Nosology in Psychiatry and Family Systems Theory

Disciplines other than medicine have also wrestled with the question of the nomenclature and classification of illness from a family or multidimensional perspective. Recent advances in psychiatry and family systems theory serve to clarify the problems which medicine currently faces as it tries to look at illness in a broader way. In the case of psychiatry, a new nosology has developed, capable of expressing several dimensions of a psychiatric problem at one time. In family systems theory, researchers are struggling to develop a typology which could classify all families, functional and dysfunctional, normal and aberrant, and which could thus serve as a basis for developing a way of describing "family illnesses," as well as for situating illness in its family context.

THE CASE OF PSYCHIATRY: DSM-III

The continuing evolution of psychiatric nosology is reflected in DSM-III, whose publication in 1980 after five years of intensive work represented a major shift in the understanding of "mental disorders." The shift is towards a phenomenological approach, which is descriptive and based on what can be observed, and thus attempts to avoid etiologically-couched diagnoses:

The approach taken in DSM-III is atheoretical with regard to etiology or pathophysiological process except for those disorders for which this is well established and therefore included in the definition of the disorder. Undoubtedly, with time, some of the disorders of unknown etiology will be found to have specific biological etiologies, others to have specific psychological causes, and still others to result mainly from a particular interplay of psychological, social, and biological factors. (DSM-III, p. 7)

One of DSM-III's main advances is the concept of *multiaxial evaluation*:

DSM-III recommends the use of a multiaxial system for evaluation to ensure that certain information that may be of value in planning treatment and predicting outcome for each individual is recorded on each of five axes, the first three of which constitute an official diagnostic evaluation. (p. 8)

All the "mental disorders" fit onto the first two axes. Axis II contains the Personality Disorders and Specific Developmental Disorders. All other clinical disorders are assigned to Axis I. This provides a way of classifying an individual's personality pattern in the presence or absence of psychiatric symptomatology, and also gives a way of listing a premorbid (contributing) personality disorder.

Axis III is reserved for all "physical disorders and conditions," such as diabetes, hypertension, inflammation of the gall bladder, and varicose veins:

The separation of this axis from the mental disorders axes is based on the tradition of separating those disorders whose manifestations are primarily behavioral or psychological (i.e. mental disorders) from those whose manifestations are not. It is necessary to have a term that can be applied to all of the disorders that are not considered "mental disorders." The phrase "organic disorder" would incorrectly imply the absence of physical factors in "mental" disorders. Hence, this manual uses the term "physical disorder," recognizing that the boundaries for these two classes of disorders . . . change as our understanding of the pathophysiology of these disorders increases. (p. 8)

DSM-III, in spite of its advances, thus holds to some fairly traditional biomedical thinking, a fact its creators fully understand. For example, its terms are focused almost exclusively on problems of the individual (identified) patient. It cannot be construed as a "systemic" approach by any stretch of the imagination.

Its final two axes are "optional," to be used in special clinical or research settings. Axis IV, Severity of Psychosocial Stressors, provides a way of integrating the psychosocial context of any mental illness. Axis V, Highest Level of Adaptive Functioning Past Year, gives a measure of the degree of a patient's incapacity and appears useful in treatment planning and predicting outcome.

Using the different DSM-III axes, one can describe the simultaneous, diverse aspects of a patient's presentation. In this sense, DSM-III deepens one's capacity to depict and appreciate the several dimensions of any ongoing, vital process.

In addition, through some new categories, DSM-III permits description of interrelationships between the "physical" and "mental" realm. For example, the category, Psychological Factors Affecting Physical Condition, "enables a clinician to note that psychological factors contribute to the initiation or exacerbation of a physical condition." This can express the emotional components of illnesses such as obesity, tension headache, ulcer, vomiting, dysmenorrhea, asthma, hypertension, colitis, and so on.

Somatoform Disorders, also a new category, includes several subtypes which express patients' neurotic fixation on somatic symptomatology, in the absence of clear-cut physical findings:

> The essential features of this group of disorders are physical symptoms suggesting physical disorder . . . for which there are no demonstrable organic findings or known physiological mechanisms and for which there is positive evidence, or a strong presumption, that the symptoms are linked to psychological factors or conflicts. (DSM-III, p. 241)

Included in this category are Somatization Disorder, known earlier as Briquet's syndrome; Conversion Disorder; Psychogenic Pain Disorder; Hypochondriasis; and Atypical Somatoform Disorder. Entering such a diagnosis on Axis II indicates that the clinician senses that most of the patient's symptoms appear to be psychological.

Finally, although it does not deal explicitly with family dynamic factors, DSM-III does provide a potential space for discussing such problems under the "V" codes. Thus one can find: V61.10 Marital problem; V61.20 Parent-child problem; and V61.80 Other specified family circumstances, as well as V62.81. Other interpersonal problem. There is even room for further psychosocial dimensions of the patient's problem, such as V62.30 Academic problem, and V62.20 Occupational problem. In other words, DSM-III provides space for the diagnosis of family, psychosocial, and developmental factors which may be associated with clinical difficulties.

This new psychiatric nosology, as we shall see, provides a model which raises questions for nosology in medicine, too. Particularly, the question of using a multiaxial nosology to deal with the multiple dimensions of illness has stirred the interest of those currently wanting to redo the medical nomenclature of diseases.

FAMILY TYPOLOGIES: KANTOR, BEAVERS, OLSON

For many years, family therapists and others have sought to describe different family types. Their assumption is that families, like individuals, come in a finite number of "types," and that these different types share dynamic patterns, problem clusters, and so on.

In psychosomatic medicine, notions of a particular personality structure for a given illness have been widely explored since the 1930s. Similarly, family therapists pursued the concept of the "schizophrenogenic family" in the 1950s and 1960s, attempting to grasp hold of that peculiar family constellation which gave rise to schizophrenic youngsters. Family nosology types, therefore, are a further outgrowth of a longstanding desire to describe typical "family-personalities."

Kantor and Lehr's description of open, closed, and random families (1975) was one of the earliest attempts to develop a family typology. Open families tended to have more permeable boundaries, more flexibility in rules, and a more democratic power structure. Closed families tended to be more rigid, more authoritarian, and more "traditional." Random families tended to be chaotic, their members disconnected.

Since then, the area of family classification has mushroomed. In recent years, presented mainly in the journal *Family Process*, two main theoretical models of the family have emerged:

1) David Olson and his co-workers (1979, 1983) have developed a Circumplex Model of Marital and Family Systems. This model takes family *cohesion* and *adaptability* as its main dimensions, but also includes family *communication* as a third critical dimension of family behavior. The authors feel these factors taken together can express the basic dynamics of family life.

Family cohesion is defined as the *emotional bonding that family members have toward one another*. Family adaptability is defined as *the ability of a marital or family system to change its power structure, role relationships, and relationship rules in response to situational and developmental stress.* Family communication is considered a "facilitating" dimension.

Taking four levels of adaptability—Rigid, Structured, Flexible, and Chaotic—as points on the vertical axis, and four levels of cohesion —Disengaged, Separated, Connected, and Enmeshed—as points along the horizontal axis, Olson develops a grid which contains 16 types of marital and family systems, e.g., Rigidly Separated, Flexibly Enmeshed, and so on (Figure 12) (Olson, Russell, and Sprenkle, 1983). He hypothesizes that the central levels of cohesion and adaptability make for optimal family functioning. The extremes are problematic.

From this model, Olson and co-workers derive a number of testable

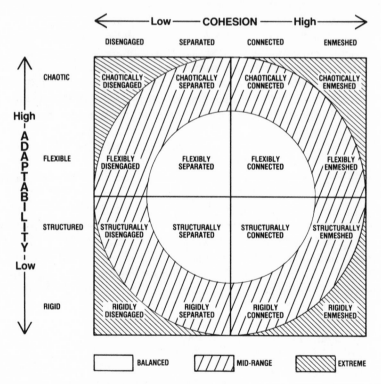

Figure 12. Circumplex Model: Sixteen Types of Marital and Family Systems.*

*Reprinted with permission from D.H. Olson, C.S. Russell, & D.H. Sprenkle, Circumplex Model of Marital and family Systems: VI. Theoretical Update, *Family Process*, 22(1), 71, 1983.

hypotheses which relate the family types to family functioning. (Further description of this topic is beyond the scope of this book. The interested reader is referred to the excellent literature in the field.)

2) W. Robert Beavers and his co-workers have developed the Beavers Systems Model (Beavers and Voeller, 1983). This is a cross-sectional model. The structure, flexibility, and competence of a family and its members are scored on one dimension and the family style on the other.

> The horizontal axis relates to the structure, available information, and adaptive flexibility of the system. In systems terms, this may be called a negentropic continuum, since the more negentropic (the more flexible and adaptive), the more the family can negotiate, function, and deal effectively with stressful situations. . . . (Beavers and Voeller, 1983, p. 89)
> The vertical axis relates to a stylistic quality of family interaction. It is . . .curvilinear. Centripetal family members view most relationship satisfaction as coming from within the family rather than from the outside world. Conversely, centrifugal family members see the outside world as holding the most promise of satisfaction and the family as holding the least. (pp. 89-91)

From this two-dimensional, "curvilinear" grid, Beavers develops nine family types, ranging from Optimal and Adequate to Midrange, and from thence to Borderline and Severely Disturbed (Figure 13).

There is essentially agreement on the dimension of cohesion with Olson's model. The difference lies in the notion of adaptability.

Olson prefers a "curvilinear" notion of adaptability, with the extremes blending into one another. Beavers views it as a linear dimension, using a "concept of systemic growth on a continuum from entropy (death of a system) to negentropy (system growth)" (Olson et al., 1983, p. 77).

Further, Beavers' notion of adaptability is represented as a "stylistic dimension" termed "centripetal/centrifugal." And:

> . . . when adaptability is seen as an emerging, ever expansible capability to be placed on a continuum ranging from dysfunctional to optimal, we have a model that is clear, coherent, and capable of integrating family systems theory with developmental theory. (Beavers and Voeller, 1983, p. 89)

These developments in family systems theory have brought thinkers closer to a common way of describing families, certainly a major devel-

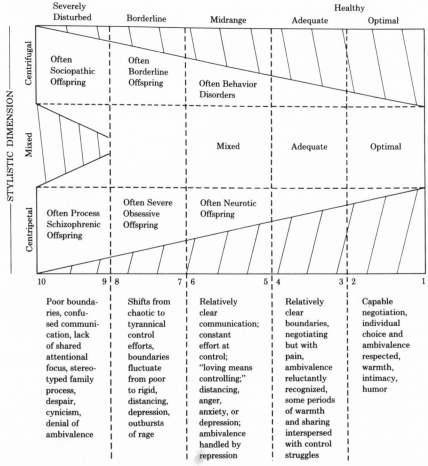

Severely Disturbed — Borderline — Midrange — Adequate — Healthy Optimal

STYLISTIC DIMENSION

Centrifugal: Often Sociopathic Offspring | Often Borderline Offspring | Often Behavior Disorders

Mixed: Mixed | Adequate | Optimal

Centripetal: Often Process Schizophrenic Offspring | Often Severe Obsessive Offspring | Often Neurotic Offspring

10	9 ¦ 8	7 ¦ 6	5 ¦ 4	3 ¦ 2	1
Poor boundaries, confused communication, lack of shared attentional focus, stereotyped family process, despair, cynicism, denial of ambivalence	Shifts from chaotic to tyrannical control efforts, boundaries fluctuate from poor to rigid, distancing, depression, outbursts of rage	Relatively clear communication; constant effort at control; "loving means controlling;" distancing, anger, anxiety, or depression; ambivalence handled by repression	Relatively clear boundaries, negotiating but with pain, ambivalence reluctantly recognized, some periods of warmth and sharing interspersed with control struggles	Capable negotiation, individual choice and ambivalence respected, warmth, intimacy, humor	

Figure 13. Beavers Systems Model.*

Autonomy: A continuous or infinite dimension, related to the family system's capacity to allow and encourage members to function competently in making choices, assuming responsibility for self, and negotiating with others.

Adaptability: A continuous or infinite dimension, related to the capacity of a family to function competently in effecting change and tolerating differentiation of members.

Centripetal/Centrifugal: A curvilinear, stylistic dimension with extreme styles associated with severely disturbed families and the most competent families avoiding either extreme.

Inflexibility: The inability to change. The most chaotic families are the most inflexible owing to their lack of a shared focus of attention.

Severely Disturbed: The lowest level of functioning along the adaptiveness continuum manifested by poorly defined subsystem boundaries and confusion owing to nonautonomous members having little tolerance for clear, responsible communication.

Borderline: A level of functioning between severely disturbed and midrange, manifested by persistent and ineffective efforts to rid the system of confusion by simplistic and often harsh efforts at control.

Midrange: Families that typically turn out sane but limited offspring, with relatively clear boundaries but continued expectations of controlling and being controlled.

*Reprinted with permission from W.R. Beavers and M.N. Voeller, Family Models: Comparing and Contrasting the Olson Circumplex Model with the Beavers Systems Model, *Family Process,* 22(1), 90, 1983.

opment for both research and clinical practice. Beavers, for example, feels that his typology is "clinically useful, empirically supported, and able to offer a valid gradation of functioning ability" (Beavers and Voeller, 1983, p. 91). This can serve as a guide to evaluating family intervention strategies, as well as to the study of normal families.

SIMILAR DEVELOPMENTS IN PRIMARY CARE*

It is not surprising that developments similar to those in psychiatry and family therapy have also occurred in primary-care nosology. The book *Psychosocial Factors Affecting Health* (1982), edited by Mack Lipkin, Jr., and Karel Kupka, traces the efforts of primary-care physicians to draft a new nosology in primary care. In this book, resulting from a 1979 conference in Washington, D.C., scholars make efforts made to develop a simple, multidimensional classification system, using preexisting classification categories wherever possible. Their work has now taken on international dimensions, leading to newly proposed ICD and ICHPPC categories.**

The new system proposes three axes, the third of which contains the family, cultural, and environmental concerns. Hyde (1983) criticizes this, pointing out the "apparent need for five rather than three axes" and commenting that DSM-III already accepts five, while the Systematized Nomenclature of Medicine works with seven axes. It is clear from his critique that the discussion among primary-care physicians is still in its early stages. Yet the general thesis, that a multidimensional nosology is needed to express what we currently understand, seems to be gaining ground. This development dovetails with the work in psychiatry and family therapy in critiquing the medical model and urging a broader, more comprehensive classification system.

---

*I am indebted to Lee Hyde (1983) for much of the information in this section.
**ICHPPC: International Classification of Health Problems in Primary Care. ICD: International Classification of Diseases.

CHAPTER 18

Summary: Towards a More Comprehensive Nosology

The breadth of scope reflected in DSM-III need not be kept limited to psychiatry. Indeed, the idea of "multiaxial" diagnosis is now challenging traditional nosology in other fields, too. Having several coexistent dimensions insures that more information will be available to the scientist-researcher; it also enables clinicians to express a broader picture of their patient's problem, as they perceive it. A multiaxial framework is thus one way to approximate the unity of the biomedical core and its psychosocial surround.

In addition, if we wish, we can use the newly developed notions of family typology as a supplement to the more traditional notions of "individual typology." That is, we can describe both the identified patient's character and the character-type of his or her family.

This would create a scheme capable of expressing many simultaneously perceived aspects of illness, in both its biomedical and its psychosocial contexts. The skeleton for such an approach is readily available now. One only has to elaborate on the model of DSM-III, adding notions of family typology.

Such a diagnosis might include statements on the following Axes:

Axis I: Physical Disorders, as in DSM-III, but on the first axis. This axis would include all of the traditional "biomedical" disorders, "physical illnesses," and the like: diabetes, ulcers, myocardial infarctions, pul-

172

monary emboli, abscesses, hyperthyroid states, brain tumors, and so on.

Axis II: Psychological Disorders felt to be present. This would be similar to DSM-III Axis I (clinical syndromes), but it could be extended to contain two subdimensions:

(a) Individual Psychological-Mental-Behavioral Disorders

(b) Disorders of Family Interaction

Axis III: Personality and Developmental Disorders. This is similar to DSM-III, Axis III, but two subdimensions can again be embraced:

(a) Individual Personality or Developmental Disorder: This can describe the personality or character type of the particular individual being discussed.

(b) Family Typology; Family Type of Developmental Disorder: This can describe, if one wishes, the "family type" of the family being discussed.

This axis can be used to express "premorbid" factors, but it would also, in some circumstances, represent the basic problem.

Axis IV: Psychosocial Factors affecting the presentation, much like DSM-III's Axis IV. This could be subdivided into Occupational, Academic, Community, etc. For example, it would address job loss; the effects of having been in a hurricane; poverty; work-related illness, such as asbestosis; etc.

Axis V: Optimal Level of Functioning in Past Year would continue to be an optional category, available for research purposes.

Diagnostic statements might look like the following (the examples are taken from my own practice):

Example 46

Judy A, age 17. This young woman has come in for treatment of diabetes. She is having a problem following her medication, and her illness is out of control. At the same time, she appears to be having troubles in school and is fighting with her parents. Suddenly, she has come in, pregnant.

Axis I.
Juvenile diabetes
Pregnancy
Axis II.
(a) Adolescent adjustment reaction
(b) ————

Axis III.
(a) Passive-aggressive personality
(b) Chaotic family
Axis IV.
Low income family; divorced mother; low level of family support
Axis V.
High school work: deteriorating grades
Held down part-time job.

Example 47

Phil B, age 27. This young man has developed an acute peptic ulcer in the context of job-related stress. In addition, he is panicked about the idea of being physically ill, and has begun having hyperventilation attacks. His marriage is under increasing strain, both from economic factors and from his physical and emotional difficulties. His wife has spoken about the possibility of a trial separation.

Axis I.
Acute peptic ulcer
Axis II.
(a) Anxiety reaction
(b) Marital discord
Axis III.
(a) Obsessional personality
(b) Centripetal, ordered nuclear family; marital pair in transition
Axis IV.
Job uncertainty
Difficulty separating from parents
Axis V.
Stable job and marriage attained in the past year.

Example 48

Molly C, age 55. This married woman with four grown children has had an exacerbation of her diabetes and hypertension, as well as her sciatic pains. She lives in a stable marriage, but her last three years have been taken up worrying over her ill mother. Because of family rivalries over who was best able to care for her mother, and repeated arguments over who mother loved best, Molly has become estranged from her brothers and sisters. She feels herself to be a martyr, unappreciated, even by her mother, and her outlook on life has darkened considerably as the months continue to drag on and her mother clings to life, demanding and shouting at Molly, while deteriorating physically to the point where she probably needs to be placed in a nursing home.

Axis I.
  Diabetes
  Sciatica
  Hypertension
Axis II.
  (a) Depression
  (b) Skewed family communication: blaming
Axis III.
  (a) Passive-aggressive personality
  (b) Matriarchal family: closed model
Axis IV.
  Financial and emotional stress of family feuding.
Axis V.
  Has managed family well for years herself.

Other examples could be given, but the idea should already be evident. The interested reader is encouraged to follow these categories to describe several patients he or she knows well and then to reflect on the information thus condensed.

CONTRA REDUCTIONISM

There are several problems with such a framework, however. The most practical one is getting any physician to fill out three, four, or five dimensions of a diagnosis. Even if clinicians accept such a framework to begin with, and even if they understand the different dimensions, writing it all down is a problem. First, it is a question of time: Many busy physicians simply will not take the necessary few minutes to write their diagnoses down in five or ten places. Diagnosis encounter sheets are already an encumbrance. To write down several disparate bits of information is perceived as an imposition. Further, physicians are often ignorant of information which would lead to a diagnosis on axes other than the biomedical.

Another problem with a multiaxial diagnostic form in medical practice is the way it presents psychological information. If the physician thinks the patient's problem is emotionally-based, but has not yet communicated this to the patient, what happens when the patient reads the record? What happens when the physician's impression is wrong and "real" illness *is* present, but he or she does not pick it up, and instead writes down that the "illness" appears to be a psychosomatic problem? This could lead to an abrupt break in the physician-patient relationship, malpractice suits, etc.

Physicians may be comfortable with thinking that a patient's "medical problem" is mainly psychosocial, but uncomfortable with putting such a view in writing. The art of medical practice has to do, in no small part, with the way a physician and his or her patient work together to develop a diagnosis. This process can be shortcircuited by a too-quick summary by the physician. In fact, the way diagnosis is often used as a reductive statement, rather than as a broadly descriptive statement, is upsetting to many of the physicians who most avidly argue for a broader notion of diagnosis.

The problem is one of reductionism, of summarizing the patient's problem in a small series of statements. Does using five statements instead of two make a diagnosis any less reductionistic? Doesn't using diagnosis this way undercut seeing the patient as a person in all his or her complexity?

More intricate diagnostic labels are not automatically good or desirable. Even if they can clarify family levels of diagnosis, their value might not outweigh their liability of reducing experience to cliché.

Many more questions arise. For example: From whose perspective is a family diagnosis made? From the physician's? From another health care provider's? From one family member's? His mother's? His son's? Does one take a consensus, or are some people's opinions more "correct" than others'? From an adolescent's point of view, a family crisis may be due to the unyielding behavior of one's neurotically rigid parents. From the parents' perspective, the problem may be a disobedient and defiant adolescent. The physician may see it as an "adolescent adjustment re-action" and identify the teenager as the "patient." The family therapist, on the other hand, may view the problem as a "developmental crisis" in a family facing abrupt transitions on many members' parts. Making every diagnosis a "developmental crisis" would be incorrect. Sometimes one area is more important—say, the parental conflict. Sometimes an-other may be—say, the teenager's personality. Sometimes both are so intimately related that one cannot tease out the two.

For this reason, premature, rigid, or automatic and unthinking di-agnoses must be avoided. A dogmatic stance, even from (especially from!) someone who pretends to be a family systems thinker, can be harmful.

Reductionism can arise in any diagnostic scheme, whether it is multiaxial, focused on family typologies, or something else. What value is
there, one can ask, in characterizing any particular family at a point in
time? Do families always stay the same type? Do they change over time?
What is gained by forcing some families into a family typology grid?
What is gained by presuming certain "basic" family typologies? Would
such typologies be culture- or class-bound, or would they exist above
the usual social parameters and determinants, crossing culture and class
lines, like Platonic ideals? Finally, do we understand enough about family types, the influence of psychosocial factors on illness, etc., to start
up a diagnostic categorization which includes them?

My sense is that such attempts at a nosology are interesting and
laudable, but premature now. Personally, I have a negative reaction to
them. I feel they are in some way squeezing the life out of the phenomenon. Instead of grasping the whole, they are still chopping it into
pieces. While giving lip-service to a "systems" approach, such schemes
as the multiaxial diagnosis act to create another linear set of parallel
categories. What is the relationship between phenomena recorded on
Axis I and those recorded on Axis II or III? The more grids, tables,
columns, and check-off spaces, the more I start to feel that the patient
gets lost, the illness gets lost, the family gets lost, and the relationship
between all these factors and the treating physician gets lost. How can
any such scheme express the dynamic, ever-changing quality of human
experience?

Developing an entire family- or systems-oriented nosology would be
valuable from a comprehensive, research-oriented viewpoint, but its
drawbacks include this temptation to cram experience into a few categories. If experience is squeezed into slots it does not easily fit, then,
it is being violated. Any proposed diagnostic schema should be used to
increase, not limit, one's understanding. It can be used if it is necessary
to obtain payment. But the thinking physician may want to avoid using
it in an automatic, dogmatic way.

DIFFERENT VIEWS

One of nosology's main purposes is to classify natural phenomena so
they can be studied and understood. Historically, there have been two
main trends regarding this task.

On the one hand, diagnostic entities have been regarded as real,
"objective things" which exist "out there" and inhabit any given patient.
(This is the gist, for example, of the ICD-9 regarding diabetes or any

other illness.) It is a view whose beginning was with Sydenham (1858), who felt that disease entities were and should be as discrete as species in the biological kingdom:

> In the first place, it is necessary that all diseases be reduced to definite and certain *species*, and that, with the same care which we see exhibited by botanists in their phytologies. . . . (Sydenham, quoted by Engle and Davis, 1963, p. 514)

A second way is to look at a diagnosis as a comprehensive description. The disease is not seen as an "entity"; yet its description is felt to be valuable to others. Such a concept has been put forth by Clark-Kennedy (1959):

> A clinical diagnosis should, wherever possible, take the form of a brief descriptive statement of your patient for the purposes of prognosis and his treatment. (p. 125)

As Engle and Davis (1963) note, however, such a definition gives "increasing recognition to the importance of individual characteristics in the formulation of a diagnosis and approach[es] the point where no two patients have precisely the same diagnosis" (p. 515).

One tendency, then, looks to develop a list of objective, predictable, recognizable illnesses. The other seeks to impart the "feel" and uniqueness of each individual patient's distress and symptomatology. The former reflects the scientific spirit, which seeks to find objective verities, definable disease categories, and distinct classifications. The second reflects the clinical stance, which seeks to discover the uniqueness of each individual patient, each individual malady: the particularity of suffering.

These are nothing less than the two great philosophical trends which have marked Western civilization for centuries: idealism, insisting on absolutes by which to measure our own mortal experience; and materialism, seeking truth in concrete experience. Objective and subjective; general and particular; eternal and time-bound, these two trends compete for dominance in the realm of diagnosis as well.

A third position also exists. This holds that diagnosis is not objective at all, but is instead an observer's convenience. Such a relativistic view refuses to take sides, and, standing above it all, says "Reality is what you say it is." This view is found among social constructivists who argue that people create their own reality, and who see diseases as one of its aspects:

In hospital jargon, "diseases" are "morbid entities" and medical students fondly believe that these "entities" somehow exist *in rebus naturae* and were discovered by their teachers much as was America by Columbus. . . . That our grouping of like cases as cases of the same disease is purely a matter of justification and convenience, liable at any moment to supersession or adjustment, is nowhere admitted; and the hope is held out that one day we shall know all the diseases that there "are" and all about them that is to be known (Crookshank, 1959, p. 342).

In fact, it may be a convenience for us to imagine that a diagnosis is a convenience. In a world where art is long and life short, we have to learn to make choices and come to conclusions. The choices any clinician faces are: 1) What ends do I want the diagnosis to serve? and 2) In what terms do I want it couched?

There is yet a fourth position, which I will call the pragmatic view. It serves physicians who have to make diagnoses in order to treat their patients. This position begins by understanding the uncertain and probabilistic nature of diagnosis. It acknowledges that diagnosis may be made on different "levels," each of which may be focused upon a different system (organ system, family, individual, etc.). It also acknowledges that the diagnosis is socially created, and that it can lay little claim to absolute objectivity. This position brings a multiplicity of factors into the diagnostic arena. Accepting a wide number of possible, simultaneous diagnostic explanations, it is able to pursue the one(s) which appears most capable of providing therapeutic assistance. At some times, the physician may explore the familial dimensions of a young girl's belly pain. At other times, he or she may pursue a medical "workup." At still other times, he may seek to minimize the whole problem and focus on something else instead. The critical difference here is that the physician is able to choose from among a wide number of possible approaches and therapeutic interventions. The physician is not, therefore, *bound* to work in any one or two ways, let us say to follow only a biomedical approach. Such a position, I would hold, is most consistent with practicing the art of clinical medicine today.

THE NOTION OF BRIGHTNESS

Pursuing the last ("fourth") perspective, diagnosis can take place at a number of different levels. At times, the biomedical level is the most appropriate (acute gall bladder attack; acutely bleeding ulcer; broken leg). At times it is not (vague abdominal pain; recurrent asthmatic attacks; palpitations due to anxiety). At times, there appear to be so many different possibilities, the clinician scarcely knows where to focus his attention.

Many "levels" of activity can be involved in any process under consideration. How does one focus on the feature which needs attention the most, which is producing the most distress, or which offers the best hope for treatment because it can best facilitate the patient or family's growth? How does a physician choose his or her point of intervention? Which factors should be pursued in the limited time available?

The concept of "brightness" provides one guide: This is an intuitive, basically visual metaphor. Simply put, the "bright" part of the system is that part filled with so much importance and energy, it would "glow" and "throb" if one put it into a dark room. Imagine that the physician could take the problem at hand—the individual in his or her network, the family system, etc.—and compact it into a globular mass. All the possible involved factors are mushed up together, rolled into a giant ball. The physician then scurries off with it to some dark closet and looks at it. Certain of its features would be glowing, pulsing with energy. In one family, with a daughter with belly pain, it would be the relationship between the daughter and her mother. In another family, whose young husband is ill with an ulcer, it would be the meaning of his tension on the job to his sense of success and failure. In another family, with an elderly aunt with a swollen leg, it would be her reluctance to take the appropriate medication, and the family's inability to set up an effective medication schedule for her. For another family, whose mother is having irregular periods, it would be making a referral for a thorough gynecological examination, before anything else. This elusive property, intuited by the physician, can be termed the "brightness" of the system. I would be the first to say this is a very unscientific concept, but it can be extremely helpful in practice. It is an excellent antidote to the obsessional listing of 300 "possibly contributing factors" by the worried and overwhelmed young physician. It means that one can use a systems approach without having to be bound by a spider web of all-the-possible-systems interlinked to one another ad infinitum, etc. When the physician feels overwhelmed by the various aspects of a complex family system, the concept of "brightness" can help him or her focus on a critical area. And such a focus is needed to provide treatment. The decisive physician cannot deal with all factors equally. Some are more worth pursuing than others. The notion of "brightness" provides a name (and therefore a legitimacy) for clinical activity which must be pursued.

CHAPTER 19

Conclusion

In the history of science, the development of theory often runs ahead of practice. New concepts appear and develop, but the old ways of dealing with problems still prevail. Practitioners resist changing their behavior, even if they feel the new ideas have merit. This is the case with medical care today.

Medical theory and research have advanced to probe implications of a systemic view of illness, but medical practice remains stuck in the biomedical model of disease. Furthermore, this model works most of the time. Most patients seeking medical care receive it, and their condition is usually made better. Yet the medical system does not examine the problems produced by its own ideology. It does not, as Antonovsky (1979) notes, explore the marvel of health, but focuses on illness instead. Nor does it look at itself as others do. Indeed, the main forces urging a reexamination of the medical model today come from outside of medicine, from people with economic considerations, or from consumer discontent.

The centerpins of the biomedical view are the twin notions of diagnosis and illness as static, linear entities. Medicine has erected a massive system around these notions, a system which is one of the most lucrative and powerful subsystems in the whole of U.S. society. This system, focused around the diagnosis and management of what it defines as "disease," has been inordinately successful, both in positioning itself

within society as a whole and in disseminating its views. From its basic
view of the physician's role, the medical system has developed several
institutions whose job is defining and treating illness.

The traditional view of illness and diagnosis has often worked well.
Yet, in many areas, especially regarding some of the most common
illnesses, the traditional view has failed to reduce mortality, prevent
sickness, or fully explain the problem. When it comes to encompassing
all that is known about illness, the traditional view is just plain inadequate. A systems approach is more satisfying, scientifically sounder. Yet
the systems approach is far from being accepted by most medical schools,
and it has made relatively few inroads on medical practice and medical
nomenclature.

Why is this so? One reason is resistance from the entrenched model
and the entrenched powers who hold it. Another reason is that the new
model has yet to convince most practicing and teaching physicians of
its value and applicability. A further obstacle has to do with the naturally
predictable resistance to any new theoretical model. Finally, people understand that it is difficult to translate the new understanding into practice. Such change involves more than simply "switching ideas." It would
involve educational, organizational, and political change. Would the
benefits justify so much effort?

I think they would. Furthermore, I think the changes wrought on
medical practice by the new theoretical model would be salutary for the
public's overall health, working to reverse the growing fragmentation
of care which has so alienated the medical consumer. Organizational
issues, however, are beyond the scope of this monograph.

I have not tried to present a solution to the problem of diagnosis, but
have attempted instead to explain the complexity and scope of the problem and its implications for clinical practice. The broader approach to
problems of clinical medicine, whether one calls it "biopsychosocial,"
"systemic," or simply "broader and deeper," heralds new responsibilities, new challenges for medicine. Many oppose such responsibilities
and prefer not to deal with the new challenges. Some current forces are
in fact successfully parlaying the traditional biomedical view of medical
care into impressive new fortunes—EmergiCenters, franchised medicine, vast groups of employed medical personnel, and so on. This effort
is so successful, in fact, that it is not at all clear that a "broader," more
humanistic version of medical care is going to survive such an assault.
If it does, it will need a new and guiding ideology, one which permits
physicians to approach patients and their illnesses in the most sophisticated, most sensitive way.

This book is written in hopes that, through advocating an approach accepting both the biomedical core and the psychosocial surround of illness phenomena, it can help influence the medical care debate of the 1980s. As Rudolf Virchow said: "Medicine is a social science, and politics is nothing more than medicine in larger scale" (1958, p. 106).

Bibliography

1. Abbott, E. A. *Flatland*. New York: Harper & Row, 1963, (1868).
2. Ader, R. *Psychoneuroimmunology*. New York: Academic Press, 1981.
3. Alexander, F. *Psychosomatic Medicine*. New York: Norton, 1932.
4. Antonovsky, A. *Health, Stress and Coping*. San Francisco: Jossey-Bass, 1979.
5. Ashby, W. R. *An Introduction to Cybernetics*. London: Chapman and Hall, 1956.
6. Auerswald, E. H. Interdisciplinary versus ecological approach. *Family Process*, 7:202-215, 1968.
7. Auerswald, E. H. The Gouverneur Health Services Program: An experiment in ecosystemic community health care delivery. *Family Systems Medicine*, 1:5-24, 1983.
8. Balint, M. *The Doctor, His Patient, and the Illness*. New York: International Universities Press, 1957.
9. Bateson, G. *Steps to an Ecology of Mind*. San Francisco: Chandler, 1972.
10. Bateson, G., Jackson, J. J., Haley, J., & Weakland, J. *Towards a theory of schizophrenia*. Behavioral Science, 1:251-269, 1956.
11. Beavers, W. R. Healthy, midrange, and severely dysfunctional families. In F. Walsh (Ed.), *Normal Family Processes*. New York: Guilford Press, 1982, pp. 45-66.
12. Beavers, W. R., and Voeller, M. N. Comparing and contrasting the Olson circumplex model with the Beavers systems model. *Family Process*, 22:85-97, 1983.
13. Bernard, C. *An Introduction to the Study of Experimental Medicine*, translated by Henry Copley Greene. New York: Dover, 1957 (1927).
14. Bibace, R. & Walsh, M. E. (Eds.). *Children's Conceptions of Health, Illness, and Bodily Functions. New Directions for Child Development #14*. San Francisco: Jossey-Bass, 1981.

15. Bowen, M. *Family Therapy in Clinical Practice*. New York: Jason Aronson, 1978.
16. Brody, H. & Waters, D. B. Diagnosis is treatment. *Journal of Family Practice*, 10:445-449, 1980.
17. Bruch, H. *Eating Disorders: Obesity, Anorexia, and the Person Within*. New York: Basic Books, 1973.
18. Buckley, W. (Ed.) *Modern Systems Research for the Behavioral Scientist*. Chicago: Aldine, 1968.
19. Bursztajn, H., Hamm, R. M., Feinbloom, R. I., & Brodsky, A. *Medical Choices, Medical Chances: How Patients, Families, and Physicians Can Cope with Uncertainty*. New York: Delacorte, 1981.
20. Cannon, W. B. *Bodily Changes in Pain, Hunger, Fear and Rage*. New York: Appleton-Century-Crofts, 1920.
21. Carmichael, L. P. Forty families—A search for the family in family medicine. *Family Systems Medicine*, 1(1):12-16, 1983.
22. Carmichael, L. P. & Carmichael, J. S. The relational model in family practice. *Marriage and Family Review*, 4:123-134, 1981.
23. Christie-Seely, J. Teaching the family concept in family medicine. *Journal of Family Practice*, 13:391-401, 1981.
24. Clark-Kennedy, A. E. *How To Learn Medicine*. London: Faber and Faber, 1959.
25. Crookshank, F. G. The importance of a theory of signs and a critique of language in the study of medicine. In C. K. Ogden & I. A. Richards (Eds.), *The Meaning of Meaning*. New York: Harcourt, Brace and World, 1959, suppl. 11.
26. Dell, P. & Goolishian, H. Order through fluctuation: An evolutionary paradigm for human systems. Presented at annual meeting of the A. K. Rice Institute. Houston, Texas, 1979.
27. *Diagnostic and Statistical Manual of Mental Disorders* (Third Edition). Washington, D.C.: American Psychiatric Association, 1980.
28. DiMatteo, M. R. & DiNicola, D. D. *Achieving Patient Compliance*. New York: Pergamon, 1982.
29. Dingle, J. H., Badger, G. F., & Jordan, W. S. *Illness in the Home*. Cleveland: Case Western Reserve University Press, 1964.
30. Doherty, W. & Baird, M. *Family Therapy and Family Medicine*. New York: Guilford Press, 1983.
31. Dubos, R. *The Mirage of Health*. New York: Harper & Row, 1979.
32. Dunbar, H. F. *Emotions and Bodily Changes: A Survey of Literature on Psychosomatic Interrelationships*. New York: Columbia University, 1954.
33. Engel, G. L. The need for a new medical model: A challenge for biomedicine. *Science*, 196:129-136, 1977.
34. Engel, G. L. The clinical application of the biopsychosocial model. *American Journal of Psychiatry*, 137:535-544, 1980.
35. Engle, R. L. Medical diagnosis: Present, past, and future. III. Diagnosis in the future, including a critique on the use of electronic computers as diagnostic aids to the physician. *Archives of Internal Medicine*, 112:530-543, 1963.
36. Engle, R. L. & Davis, B. J. Medical diagnosis: Present, past, and future.

I. Present concepts of the meaning and limitations of medical diagnosis. *Archives of Internal Medicine*, 112:512-519, 1963.

37. Feinstein, A. R. *Clinical Judgment*. Baltimore: Williams & Wilkins, 1967.
38. Fleck, S. Family functioning and family pathology. *Psychiatric Annals*, 10:46-57, 1980.
39. Foucault, M. *Madness and Civilization: A History of Insanity in the Age of Reason*. New York: Random House, 1965.
40. Fox, R. C. The medicalization and demedicalization of American society. *Daedelus*, 106:9-22, 1977.
41. Freidson, E. *Profession of Medicine: A Study of the Sociology of Applied Knowledge*. New York: Harper & Row, 1970.
42. Friedman, M. *Pathogenesis of Coronary Artery Disease*. New York: McGraw-Hill, 1969.
43. Garner, A. & Weinar, C. *The Mother-Child Interaction in Psychosomatic Disorders*. Urbana: University of Illinois Press, 1959.
44. Gerson, E. M. The social character of illness—Deviance or politics? *Social Science and Medicine*, 10:219-224, 1976.
45. Goldberg, E. M. *Family Influences of Psychosomatic Illness*. London: Tavistock, 1958.
46. Grolnick, L. A family perspective of psychosomatic factors in illness. *Family Process*, 11:457-486, 1972.
47. Hall, A. & Fagen, R. Definition of a system. In B. D. Ruben & J. Y. Kim (Eds.), *General Systems Theory and Human Communication*. Rochelle Park, NJ: Hayden, 1978.
48. Henderson, L. J. Physician and patient as a social system. *New England Journal of Medicine*, 212:819-823, 1935.
49. Hingson, R., Scotch, N. A., Sorenson, J., & Swazey, J. P. *In Sickness and in Health: Social Dimensions of Medical Care*. St. Louis: C. V. Mosby, 1981.
50. Hippocrates. Cambridge, MA: Loeb Classical Library, trans. W. H. S. Jones, 1923 (1972).
51. Hoffman, L. *Foundations of Family Therapy*. New York: Basic Books, 1981.
52. Huygen, F. J. A. *Family Medicine: The Medical Life History of Families*. New York: Brunner/Mazel, 1982.
53. Huygen, F. J. A. & Smits, A. J. A. Family therapy, family somatics, and family medicine. *Family Systems Medicine*, 1:23-32, 1983.
54. Hyde, L. Book Review. *Family Systems Medicine*, 1(4):94-97, 1983.
55. Hyde, L. Family work: A nosology and approach to family tasks and problems with the language of family medicine, a draft vocabulary. Unpublished manuscript, 1984.
56. Illich, I. *Medical Nemesis: The Expropriation of Health*. New York: Pantheon, 1976.
57. Kanner, L. Children as organs of parental hypochondriasis. *Child Psychiatry*, 616, 1948.
58. Kantor, D. & Lehr, W. *Inside the Family*. San Francisco: Jossey-Bass, 1975.
59. Kellner, R. *Family Ill Health: An Investigation in General Practice*. New York: Charles C. Thomas, 1963.
60. Klein, R., Dean, A., & Bogdanoff, M. The impact of illness upon the spouse. *Journal of Chronic Diseases*, 20:241-252, 1968.

61. Kraus, A. S. & Lilienfield, A. M. Some epidemiological aspects of the high mortality rate in the young widowed group. *Journal of Chronic Diseases*, 10:207-215, 1959.
62. Kreitman, N. The patient's spouse. *British Journal of Psychiatry*, 110:159-167, 1964.
63. Laszlo, E. *The Systems View of the World*. New York: George Braziller, 1972.
64. Levy, R. L. The role of social support in patient compliance: A selective review. In *Patient compliance to prescribed antihypertensive medication regimes* (Dept. HEW, PHS, NIH Publication #81-2102). Washington, D.C.: U.S. Government Printing Office, 1980.
65. Lipkin, M. & Kupka, K. (Eds). *Psychosocial Factors Affecting Health*. New York: Praeger, 1983.
66. Lipowski, S. J., Lipsitt, D. R., & Whybrow, P. C. (Eds.). *Psychosomatic Medicine*. New York: Oxford University Press, 1977.
67. Locke, S. E. Stress, adaptation, and immunity. *General Hospital Psychiatry*, 4:49-58, 1982.
68. Lynch, J. J. *The Broken Heart: Medical Consequences of Loneliness*. New York: Basic Books, 1979.
69. MacKinnon, R. A. & Michels, R. *The Psychiatric Interview in Clinical Practice*. Philadelphia: W. B. Saunders, 1971.
70. *A Manpower Policy for Primary Health Care*. Washington, D.C.: National Academy of Sciences, 1978.
71. Mao Tse-tung. *On Contradiction*. Peking: Foreign Languages Press, 1966.
72. Mechanic, D. *Medical Sociology*. New York: Macmillan, 1978.
73. Medalie, J. M. Introductory remarks. *The Family in Family Medicine: Present State and Future Trends*. Conference. Ann Arbor, Michigan, June 18, 1982.
74. Medalie, J. M., Snyder, M., Groen, J. J., et al. Angina pectoris among 10,000 men: Five year incidence and univariate analysis. *American Journal of Medicine*, 55:583, 1973.
75. Meissner, W. W. Family dynamics and psychosomatic processes. *Family Process*, 5:142-161, 1966.
76. Meyer, R. J. & Haggerty, R. J. Streptococcal infections in families: Factors altering individual susceptibility. *Pediatrics*, 29:539-549, 1962.
77. Minuchin, S., Montalvo, B., Guerney, B. G., Rosman, B. L., & Schumer, F. *Families of the Slums: An Exploration of Their Structure and Treatment*. New York: Basic Books, 1967.
78. Minuchin, S., Rosman, B. L., & Baker, L. *Psychosomatic Families*. Cambridge: Harvard University Press, 1978.
79. Mishler, E. G., AmaraSingham, L. R., Hauser, S. T., Liem, R., Osherson, S. D., & Waxler, N. E. *Social Contexts of Health, Illness, and Patient Care*. Cambridge: Cambridge University Press, 1981.
80. Obituary of M. Balint. *International Journal of Psychoanalysis*, 52:332-333, 1971.
81. Olson, D. H., Russell, C. S., & Sprenkle, D. H. Circumplex model of marital and family systems: VI. Theoretical update. *Family Process*, 22:69-83, 1983.
82. Olson, D. H., Sprenkle, D. H., & Russell, C. S. Circumplex model of marital and family systems: I. Cohesion and adaptability dimensions, family types, and clinical applications. *Family Process*, 18:3-28, 1979.
83. Patterson, J. M. Remarks. *The Family in Family Medicine*. Spring Conference, Society of Teachers of Family Medicine, Kansas City, March 1983.

84. Parkes, C. M. Effects of bereavement on physical and mental health: A study of the medical records of widows. *British Journal of Medicine*, 2:274-279, 1964.
85. Parkes, C. M. *Bereavement: Studies of Grief in Adult Life*. New York: International Universities Press, 1972.
86. Parsons, T. *The Social System*. New York: Free Press, 1951.
87. Peachey, R. Family patterns of stress. *General Practitioner*, 27:82-89, 1963.
88. Pepper, S. C. *World Hypotheses: A Study in Evidence*. Berkeley: University of California Press, 1942.
89. Ransom, D. C. Personal communication, 1982.
90. Ransom, D. C. On why it is useful to say that "the family is a unit of care" in family medicine: Comment on Carmichael's essay. *Family Systems Medicine* 1(1):17-23, 1983a.
91. Ransom, D. C. Random notes: The family as patient—What does this mean? *Family Systems Medicine*, 1(2):99-103, 1983b.
92. Ransom, D. C. Random notes: The family as patient—Part II. *Family Systems Medicine*, 1(3):110-113, 1983c.
93. Rees, W. D. & Lutkins, G. S. Mortality of bereavement. *British Medical Journal*, 4:13-20, 1967.
94. Richardson, H. B. *Patients Have Families*. New York: Commonwealth Fund, 1948.
95. Rosenbaum, M. (Ed.). *Compliant Behavior: Beyond Obedience to Authority*. New York: Human Sciences Press, 1983.
96. Rosenblatt, R. A., Cherkin, D. C., Schneeweiss, R., et al. The structure and content of family practice: Current status and future trends. *Journal of Family Practice*, 15:681, 1982.
97. Schmidt, D. D. The family as the unit of medical care. *Journal of Family Practice*, 7:303-313, 1978.
98. Segall, A. The sick role concept: Understanding illness behavior. *Journal of Health and Social Behavior*, 17:163-170, 1976.
99. Selye, H. *The Stress of Life*. New York: McGraw-Hill, 1956.
100. Socrates. In K. R. Pelletier, *Mind as Healer, Mind as Slayer*. New York: Dell, 1977, p. 156.
101. Stephens, G. G. *The Intellectual Basis of Family Practice*. Tucson: Winter Publishing Company, 1982.
102. Stoeckle, J. D. & Barsky, A. J. Attributions: Uses of social science knowledge in the "doctoring" of primary care. In L. Eisenberg & A. Kleinman (Eds.), *The Relevance of Social Science for Medicine*. Boston: D. Reidel, 1980, pp. 223-240.
103. Sullivan, H. S. *The Interpersonal Theory of Psychiatry*. New York: W. W. Norton, 1953.
104. Sydenham, T. *The Works of Thomas Syndenham, M.D.* Translated by R. G. Latham. London: The Sydenham Society, 1858.
105. Sylvius. In E. H. Ackerknecht, *A Short History of Medicine* (Revised edition). Baltimore: Johns Hopkins University Press, 1982, pp. 121-124.
106. Szasz, T. S. *The Myth of Mental Illness*. New York: Harper & Row, 1974.
107. Szasz, T. S. & Hollander, M. H. A contribution to the philosophy of medicine. *Archives of Internal Medicine*, 97:585-592, 1956.
108. Twaddle, A. C. The concepts of the sick role and illness behavior. *Advances*

in *Psychosomatic Medicine*, 8:162-179, 1972.
109. Virchow, R. *Disease, Life, and Man*. Translated by L. J. Rather. Stanford: Stanford University Press, 1958.
110. von Bertalanffy, L. *General System Theory*. New York: Braziller, 1968.
111. Waitzkin, H. & Stoeckle, J. D. Information control and the micropolitics of health care: Summary of an ongoing research project. *Social Science and Medicine*, 10:263-276, 1976.
112. Walsh, F. (Ed.) *Normal Family Processes*. New York: Guilford Press, 1982.
113. Watzlawick, P., Beavin, J., & Jackson, D. D. *Pragmatics of Human Communication*. New York: W. W. Norton, 1967.
114. Watzlawick, P., Weakland, J. H., & Fisch, J. R. *Change: Principles of Problem Formation and Problem Resolution*. New York: Norton, 1974.
115. Weakland, J. H. Family somatics—A neglected edge. *Family Process*, 16:263-272, 1977.
116. *Webster's Third New International Dictionary*, Unabridged. Springfield, MA: G. & C. Merriam, 1981, p. 1117.
117. Widmer, R. B., Cadoret, R. J., & North, C. S. Depression in family practice: Some effects in spouses and children. *Journal of Family Practice*, 10:45-51, 1980.
118. Worby, C. The family in the undergraduate medical school curriculum. Keynote address, Society of Teachers of Family Medicine Spring Conference, Kansas City, February 12, 1980.
119. Young, M., Benjamin, B., & Walks, C. Mortality of widowers. *Lancet*, 2:454, 1963.
120. Zola, I. K. Culture and symptoms: An analysis of patients' presenting complaints. *American Sociological Review*, 31:615-630, 1966.
121. Zola, I. K. *Socio-Medical Inquiries: Recollections, Reflections, and Reconsiderations*. Philadelphia: Temple University Press, 1983.

Name Index

191

On Diagnosis

Subject Index